the
emotional wellness
way to
cardiac health

How Letting Go

of Depression,

Anxiety & Anger

Can Heal

Your Heart

ARTHUR M. NEZU, PH.D., ABPP
CHRISTINE MAGUTH NEZU, PH.D., ABPP
DIWAKAR JAIN, MD, FRCP

New Harbinger Publications, Inc.

Distributed in Canada by Raincoast Books

Copyright © 2005 by Arthur M. Nezu, Christine Maguth Nezu, and Diwakar Jain
New Harbinger Publications, Inc.
5674 Shattuck Avenue
Oakland, CA 94609

Cover design by Amy Shoup
Acquired by Spencer Smith
Text design by Tracy Marie Carlson

ISBN 1-57224-374-0 Paperback
Library of Congress Cataloging in Publication Data on file

New Harbinger Publications' Web site address: www.newharbinger.com

07   06   05

10   9   8   7   6   5   4   3   2   1

First printing

To hope, courage, and gratitude

Contents

Part 3
Coping with Negative Emotions

Preface

Did you know that depression is fairly common among people with various types of heart disorders? Not just feelings of sadness or being "down," which would be expected of anyone experiencing a major illness, but clinical levels of depression. How common? Very common. For example, approximately two in five patients newly diagnosed with coronary heart disease (CHD) are depressed (Wulsin and Singal 2003). Moreover, depression is associated with increased cardiac illness and death in people with CHD, especially following an acute heart attack. Thus, depression can play a major role in the prognosis for a heart patient. In other words, if a heart patient is depressed (regardless of whether the person admits to it), his or her prognosis is significantly less optimistic compared to the heart patient who is not depressed. In fact, among initially disease-free individuals, depression has been found to actually increase the risk for developing CHD (Wulsin and Singal 2003).

The important association between negative emotional states, such as depression, anxiety, and anger, and cardiovascular disease, including CHD and myocardial infarctions (heart attacks), and difficulties with the heart's electric system, such as ventricular tachycardia, has been identified in scientific study after scientific study. These are not pseudoscientific or New Age speculations. The vast majority of this type of research is published in prestigious medical and psychological journals.

It is because the association between negative emotions and heart disease is not well publicized, despite decades of research, that we decided to write this book. Although the exact role that psychological variables play in causing heart disease remains somewhat controversial among the entire medical community, no health professional will argue that emotional well-being is counter to a healthy heart. In fact, the premise of this book, based on a large body of scientific literature, is that a healthy mind and a healthy emotional state can have a positive effect on your heart's physical health. So read on—find out how you can more effectively address important "matters of the heart."

It is one thing for a health professional to provide you with global advice, no matter how sound, such as "Reduce your stress" or "Eat better," but quite a different thing for you to actually know how to accomplish such goals. One of the things you may think when getting such advice is *Easy for you to say, hard for me to do!* That's why, rather than simply suggesting a list of actions you should take in order to cope with negative emotions, we will offer lots of very specific steps to help improve your overall emotional well-being.

In this book, we provide ways for you to determine whether you are experiencing any significant symptoms of emotional distress, learn a wide range of strategies that can help you overcome such symptoms, and engage in an emotional lifestyle that can improve your overall well-being, both psychologically and physically.

We certainly are not saying that such help will take the place of other sound medical advice about your health, such as eating less fatty foods and exercising more. Rather, we wrote this book to serve as part of a comprehensive plan concerning a heart-healthy lifestyle.

We wish to acknowledge the support of Spencer Smith at New Harbinger, who made this a reality; the copyediting genius of Jessica Beebe; the aid of our graduate students and fellows at Drexel; and the courage of the multitude of heart patients with whom we have worked over the years.

—Arthur M. Nezu, Ph.D.
—Christine Maguth Nezu, Ph.D.
—Diwakar Jain, M.D.

Part I

The Mind-Heart Connection

1

Why You Should Read This Book

Chances are you picked up this book for one of the following reasons:

Your cardiologist has suggested that you seek help in managing negative feelings, such as depression, anxiety, or anger because he or she believes that such distress can have an adverse impact on your current heart condition. If so, you are similar to John, a fifty-one-year-old accountant who is recovering from a heart attack. He became depressed when he lost his job eighteen months ago and continued to have problems getting a new job. John has a history of heart problems and tends to react strongly when under stress. His cardiologist recommended that he seek counseling because his depression became more intense after the heart attack. Although John feels grateful that he survived the crisis, he continues to feel hopeless about the future, especially as debts rise and his oldest son is due to go to college in a year. A heart attack plus depression can potentially be a lethal combination. John's doctor knows that scientific research shows that clinical depression has been associated with a fourfold increase in the risk of death during the first six months following an acute heart attack (Frasure-Smith, Lespérance, and Talajic 1993). John's doctor hoped that by recommending counseling to John as a means of reducing his depression, this patient might also decrease the risk of further complications and heart problems.

You have been told that you are at significant risk for a heart attack, and among other life changes (for example, losing weight or stopping smoking), you were told

to stop getting so angry at people. If so, you are similar to Mary, a forty-four-year-old widow and mother of three children. Although she makes a decent salary as the manager of a sporting goods store, she continues to find it difficult to save money. Her major "stress busters," according to her, are smoking cigarettes and eating snacks while watching movies with her kids. When we first met her, Mary candidly told us she realized that she needed to stop smoking and to revise her diet, as she had gained close to twenty-five pounds in the two years after her husband died. Moreover, she admitted that during her checkup with her primary care physician, she had to face the idea that she frequently got angry at her kids and especially with people at work. "I sometimes feel like my head is going to explode," she explained. Believing that only men are vulnerable to heart disease, she never thought about the possibility that she might develop heart problems. An annual physical exam required by her employer's medical insurance program was an eye-opener to her, especially because she was starting to experience breathing problems, fatigue, and lack of energy. Her physician suggested that she talk to a psychologist to learn anger management techniques and develop a happier and more heart-healthy lifestyle, which would also include quitting smoking and losing some weight.

Having recently had a heart attack or other cardiovascular problem, you are feeling down and somewhat hopeless and simply want to feel better. If so, you might easily relate to Paul, a forty-nine-year-old cook. Although an implantable cardioverter defibrillator (ICD) operation was successful and is highly likely to prevent sudden cardiac death, Paul continues to feel depressed months after his medical recovery. Paul's medical prognosis is good, but he feels very restricted in his activities. He had to stop coaching the local Little League baseball team; he feels he is always burdening his wife, Elsa, especially since he began to feel nervous about driving and now has her drive him to work and back; and he is generally depressed. Although he knows that depression could worsen his heart problems, he is more concerned about his overall quality of life. When we first met him, he lamented, "Even if I get to live a long time now with the ICD helping me, what kind of life is this, being down all the time? I just don't feel hopeful about the future, and I know I bring my wife down as well. Can you help me feel better? What can I do to get myself out of the dumps?"

We told him that simultaneously experiencing both medical and emotional difficulties can put a major strain on anyone's life, but improving overall emotional well-being is an important goal by itself. Gro Harlem Brundtland, the director-general of the World Health Organization, predicted that by the year 2020, the three leading causes of death or disability across all age groups around the world, barring any unexpected new communicable diseases, will be heart disease, mental depression, and road accidents (1999). This prediction suggests that we are all paying less attention to our mental and emotional health than we should. It was good to see that Paul was motivated to overcome his distress and negative emotions.

You recently read in a magazine that reducing emotional distress can actually improve a heart patient's prognosis. If so, you are similar to Karen, a forty-four-year-old office manager who is interested in maintaining a heart-healthy lifestyle. She generally exercises, eats a balanced diet, and practices yoga routinely. She is always interested in learning new ways to better manage stress and maintain balance in her life. She frequently reads magazine and newspaper articles on lifestyle and health, and she attends health fairs and conferences open to the general public. It was at one of these events, where we were presenting a stress management workshop, that we met Karen. In fact, it was people like Karen, who asked if there was a book on the market for the public about emotions and cardiac health, who actually spurred us on to write this very book.

In essence, we believe in the adage "An ounce of prevention is worth a pound of cure." Football fans will be familiar with another saying: "The best defense is a good offense." In chapter 3, we'll discuss a variety of risk factors for various cardiovascular diseases, including excess weight, high blood cholesterol, and tobacco use. In chapters 4, 5, and 6, we'll discuss how psychological factors such as depression, anxiety, and anger can also be potential risk factors for heart problems.

Never smoking can serve to reduce your risk for heart disease. If you currently smoke, it is a sound decision to stop as one way to reduce such a risk. Similarly, you can reduce your risk of poor cardiovascular health by improving your overall emotional well-being and ability to adapt to stress. Improving your overall emotional well-being is a worthwhile defense against this type of risk.

You are a friend or a family member of someone with heart disease. If so, then you might be like Martha, the sixty-two-year-old wife of Arnold, who just came out of a cardiac rehab program. Although Arnold, who is sixty-six, tends to be very interested in doing what he can to maintain his health, Martha feels that he is a bit lazy and needs some prodding. In particular, she noticed that two months after his "graduation" from rehab, Arnold engages in very few of the exercises and activities that were prescribed for him. Martha also noticed that Arnold was getting more and more nervous each day. He seemed to feel that if he exerted himself, he would have another heart attack. Wanting him to have as full a life as possible, Martha contacted us for advice. Our goal was to help Arnold reduce his overall stress and improve his emotional well-being. We prescribed several of the techniques described in this book, and we taught many to Martha as well so she could serve as a friendly coach to Arnold. In our work with cancer patients, we have found that having a spouse or partner be involved to this extent significantly increases the positive impact of counseling (Nezu et al. 2003).

WHY YOU SHOULD BE CONCERNED ABOUT YOUR EMOTIONAL HEALTH

Even if your situation mirrors that of one of the people mentioned above, you might still be asking, *Why should I read this book? I can't help that I'm under so much stress! After all, I'm not crazy or anything like that. I'm concerned about my heart, not my mind or my emotions.*

Even if you have such thoughts, before you put this book down, read the following:

- A study conducted by researchers at Harvard found that a more optimistic outlook in older men was linked with a dramatically reduced risk of CHD (Kubzansky et al. 2001).

- A research article in the prestigious journal *Circulation*, published by the American Heart Association, described a nine-year study where investigators concluded that reducing emotional distress through a rehabilitation program improved the prognosis of 150 men with CHD (Denollet and Brutsaert 2001).

- The National Heart Foundation of Australia, after reviewing the body of scientific research examining the relationship between stress and CHD, concluded in a recent position paper that "there is strong and consistent evidence of an independent causal association between depression, social isolation, and lack of quality social support and the causes and prognosis of CHD" (Bunker et al. 2003, p. 272). Note the word "independent," which indicates that these psychological and social factors can lead to CHD by themselves.

- One recent review of the scientific literature, entitled "Do Depressive Symptoms Increase the Risk for the Onset of Coronary Disease?" concluded that depressive symptoms not only contribute to a significant and independent (note the word "independent" again) risk for the onset of heart disease but actually pose a greater risk than that associated with secondhand smoke (Wulsin and Singal 2003).

- A recent study of 812 employees at a company in the Finnish metal industry, all of whom were free from cardiovascular disease at the beginning of the study, found that at a ten-year follow-up evaluation, employees with high job strain (defined as high work demands coupled with low job control) had a 200 percent higher risk for death from a cardiovascular disease than their colleagues with low job strain (Kivimäki et al. 2002).

- A study investigating the role of anger found that among 1,623 patients who previously suffered a heart attack, the risk of another heart attack after an episode of anger was increased by 200 percent (Mittleman et al. 1995).

- Many studies also demonstrate the importance of social support. For example, Berkman, Leo-Summers, and Horwitz (1992) found a three-fold increase in subsequent cardiac events among a sample of post–heart attack patients who reported a low level of emotional support. Similarly, Williams, Barefoot, and Califf (1992) observed a 300 percent increase in the likelihood of death among patients with CHD who were unmarried or without a significant relationship.

■ Life-threatening *ventricular arrhythmias* (that is, abnormal heartbeats or rhythms) appear to occur not randomly but in a pattern that suggests a relationship with the beginning and end of the workweek, independent of the influence of age, gender, type of heart disease, and use of heart medication (Peters et al. 1996).

All these studies, and hundreds of others, strongly point to a significant link between a variety of psychosocial factors and cardiovascular disease. Because of such scientific findings, it is important to be concerned about how your emotional life affects your cardiovascular health, whether you currently have heart disease or not. In other words, it is important to "mind your heart."

How Your Mind Affects Your Heart

You or a friend have probably experienced the following scenario. You know a couple who are very much in love with each other, are very close, and have a strong and longtime relationship. Unfortunately, one of them passes away. Regardless of the reason for the death, you and your friends are not surprised when the other person of this committed couple passes away soon after. You may think that the second person "died of a broken heart." You probably don't mean this literally, but you do feel that a strong sense of sadness had a negative effect on that person's overall health, even to the extent that the person died from this sadness.

If you believe in a strong mind-body connection—a strong and reciprocal relationship between how we think, feel, and act and our physical health—the basic notion behind this book will not be surprising at all. In fact, this perspective is rather old. Consider this quote from the sixteenth-century physician Phillippus Paracelsus, known as the father of modern pharmacology and credited with helping to create modern medicine: "The power of the imagination is a great factor in medicine. It may produce diseases in man ... and it may cure them." Consider also this quote by eighteenth-century philosopher Anacharsis Cloots: "Bad mind, bad heart." Lastly, consider the role that Martin Luther suggested spirituality plays in health: "Heavy thoughts bring on physical maladies; when the soul is oppressed, so is the body." So, such a belief—that the mind and body are closely tied with each other—has been around for centuries.

However, it has only been since the second half of the twentieth century that various disciplines within scientific and medical research and practice have focused on the integration of psychosocial and somatic aspects of health. These include the fields of behavioral medicine, psychosomatic medicine, and health psychology (see Nezu, Nezu, and Geller 2003 for a comprehensive overview of these areas). The essence of these fields is their adoption of a *biopsychosocial* model of disease, illness, health, and wellness. Simply put, this model suggests that biological, psychological, and social factors all represent crucial aspects of the cause, course, prognosis, and treatment of disease. During the past several decades, efforts by a wide range of health professionals, including physicians, psychologists, nurses, and research scientists, have provided substantial support of this model.

How the Mind Affects Heart Disease

In chapters 4, 5, and 6, when we discuss the relationship between various negative emotions and heart disease, we will provide more details about some of the biological mechanisms of action (that is, the biological reasons why emotions and heart disease are related). But here are some examples:

- *Heart rate variability* (HRV) is the regulation of the *sinoatrial node,* or natural pacemaker of the heart, by the autonomic nervous system (we'll discuss the autonomic nervous system in chapter 3). Reduced HRV has been found to be a strong predictor of mortality in patients who recently experienced a heart attack. Further, studies are finding a strong link between reduced HRV and depression (Carney et al. 2002), suggesting a link between depression and heart disease. Therefore, being depressed can actually enhance the heart's *arrhythmogenic potential* (that is, increase the risk for problems with the heart's rhythms; Rozanski, Blumenthal, and Kaplan 1999).

- Chronic and acute life stress can lead to elevated arterial blood pressure; acute stress can induce *myocardial ischemia* (that is, blockage of the coronary arteries that results in insufficient blood and oxygen getting to the heart). For example, recalling past events that have made you angry can actually trigger myocardial ischemia (Mittleman et al. 1995).

- Mental stress can decrease the electrical stability of the heart, which can lead to the development of arrhythmias and sudden cardiac death (Lown, Verrier, and Rabinowitz 1977).

FREQUENTLY ASKED QUESTIONS ABOUT DISTRESS

You may now be more convinced that there is a strong mind-body connection between negative emotions and heart disease, but you still may have some questions about feeling distressed. The following are common questions that heart patients have asked us in the past.

I had my heart attack at a time when I wasn't upset. How can stress and heart problems be related? People usually don't have heart attacks immediately after eating a high-fat meal either. It is the cumulative effect of stress that is responsible for the link between negative emotions and heart disease.

If I'm experiencing some emotional difficulties, such as depression or anxiety, does that mean I'm crazy? Of course not! We all experience stress. Sometimes stress is a good thing when it helps energize us to do a better job or makes us alert. Many times, however, stress can be excessive and can lead to negative physical and emotional symptoms. Some people have never learned effective ways of dealing with this stress. That's what this book, in large part, is all about—learning ways to cope with the stresses of life, especially those connected with having a heart problem.

Experiencing negative stress symptoms, like depression, anxiety, headaches, or pain, is your body's way of telling you that something is going on and that you need to do something differently. It's like a red stop sign telling you to stop.

When people use the word "crazy," they are usually referring to a condition where a person loses touch with reality and therefore loses the ability to function adequately on a day-to-day basis. Being depressed or anxious does not mean that at all. At times, people who experience depression or anxiety might feel as if they are losing control, but that is much different than actually losing touch with reality.

Experiencing negative physical and emotional symptoms simply means that you are human and not a robot. Some people may try to deny or avoid such feelings because they are concerned about being crazy or weak or a burden to others. Unfortunately, that's like a woman denying the existence of a lump in her breast or a man ignoring occasional minor chest pains. Both situations may turn out to be benign—or they can be quite serious. Using this guidebook may be of significant help. But you won't know until you try it. It's a good idea not to bury your head in the sand.

If I have problems, does that mean that I'm a failure or have a weak character? Experiencing emotional distress has nothing to do with being a failure or having a weak character. Depression, anxiety, and other emotional difficulties are caused by the complex interplay among various genetic, biological, psychological, and social factors. Some people have biological or physical vulnerabilities to emotional problems. Others may never have learned how to successfully deal with stress and therefore experience uncomfortable feelings or sad thoughts. Many times, the stress gets too overwhelming and usual ways of coping don't work. The notion that only weak people experience emotional problems is simply a myth. Depression and anxiety are very common problems. Unfortunately, this type of belief can prevent you from seeking help or doing something about a problem. Going down that road just makes things worse. Actually, facing up to your problems takes strength. To think that being depressed or anxious is weak is to call people like Martin Luther, Vincent van Gogh, Ernest Hemingway, Patty Duke, Mike Wallace, and Abraham Lincoln failures because they experienced such symptoms.

If I do seek help, how do I know it's going to be effective? All of the advice contained in this book is based on years of sound scientific research and expert clinical experience. We offer specific self-help strategies and tools that are well documented as effective counseling and psychotherapy treatment approaches. Following the advice in this book (in consultation with your physician, psychologist, or counselor when necessary) can put you on the road to successfully achieving your goals. You can learn to change the way you think, feel, and behave to reach these goals.

I've already read many of these self-help guidebooks. Why is this one any better? Most importantly, we wrote this book with the heart patient in mind. Although many of the tools contained in this book can be very effective for patients experiencing other medical problems (as we know from our research with cancer patients as well as those with other physical problems; Nezu et al. 1998; Nezu, Nezu, and Lombardo 2001), we developed this guidebook based on our years of experience with heart patients.

Many of the other self-help books found in your local bookstore are based on the latest fad, with little scientific evidence to support their effectiveness. In addition, many of these guidebooks are based on a single theory or on the author's experience. We have been careful to include a wide range of effective strategies based on hundreds of scientific studies. We believe in the old saying "Different strokes for different folks." Not everyone who uses this guide will find each tool to be helpful or useful for his or her own problems or circumstances. That's why we include many different tools to choose from. We realize that you are an individual and can be very different from another person, even if that other person is experiencing the same heart problem. So, we developed this collection of self-help strategies to keep your uniqueness in mind and not treat you like just another patient.

HOW THIS BOOK CAN HELP YOU

This book provides a tool chest of self-help strategies that can help you effectively manage and overcome those negative emotions—including depression, anxiety, and anger—that have been found to have a significant relationship to a variety of cardiovascular disorders, including coronary heart disease and problems with the heart's electrical system (for example, ventricular tachycardia and sudden cardiac death). By improving your emotional well-being, it is possible that you can improve your physical health as well and actually prevent negative emotions from having any effect on your heart health.

In the next chapter, you will have the opportunity to evaluate whether you are experiencing symptoms of depression, anxiety, or anger. Based on this assessment, we will provide you with instructions on how best to use this book. In chapter 2, we describe several different types of self-help strategies, including thinking tools, behavioral action tools, and relaxation tools. Some tools are more appropriate for certain problems or for certain people. We do not assume that everyone is exactly the same; that's why we provide a wide variety of strategies. Also in chapter 2, you will learn which type of strategy might best suit you. However, just as few people only like one flavor of ice cream, you will probably find yourself using a variety of the tools included in this book rather than just one.

In chapter 3, we offer a brief primer about the heart and heart disease.

In part 2, we include three separate chapters that address depression, anxiety, and anger and the relationship of each to cardiovascular disease. In addition, we will describe the symptoms of each emotional problem and help you determine if you are experiencing any symptoms that may affect your health. We will also note which of the self-help tools is better suited for which type of problem.

The remainder of the book, part 3, includes fourteen different chapters that describe a multitude of tools, all of which have been shown, through scores of scientific studies, to have a positive impact on overall stress and emotional distress and to improve one's quality of life. It is not necessary to read each chapter; again, not all people will find all the tools helpful. But we have come across few patients who did not benefit from most of them.

Read on! We wish you the best in taking care of your mind, your emotions, and your heart.

2

How to Assess
Your Needs

We have written this self-help book specifically for heart patients who are interested in improving their overall emotional well-being. Unlike other self-help guides, this book doesn't have to be read in its entirety. Depending on the results from the tests that you will take in this chapter, you will be directed toward certain parts. On the other hand, if you simply want to know more, feel free to read any section that interests you. Most people are likely to benefit from reading the entire book, but we structured it so that you can use it to best meet your own needs.

We will give you direct and specific advice on how to deal with your difficulties. Your goals might be to decrease your depression, improve your relationships, or overcome some anxiety. We will describe in detail many strategies that you can use to achieve such goals. These self-help tools are based on years of scientific research and clinical practice. They have proved effective in helping others, and they can be of help to you.

HOW TO USE THIS BOOK

You don't have to read this book from cover to cover. But to be able to use this book effectively, you need to read this chapter carefully. In this chapter, you will learn how to navigate through the book to obtain the best advice efficiently and in a way that is specific to you.

Part 2 of this book, "Understanding Your Emotions," provides information about three sets of negative emotions, each of which has been identified as an important risk factor for heart disease: depression, anxiety and stress, and anger and hostility. Later in this chapter, you will be asked to take a test to help you identify which of these three chapters is important for you to read in detail. We'll help you assess your feelings and determine what your scores reveal about your current emotional well-being. Your scores will show you which goals you need to set at this time: to decrease your depression, decrease your anxiety, or better manage your anger.

Based on your goals, part 3 helps to answer the question *How can I improve my emotional well-being?* Specifically, this section contains fourteen different tools to help you better manage negative emotions in order to be more heart-healthy. Each strategy is described in user-friendly terms and explained step-by-step. Later in this chapter, we will help you to answer a second important question: *How do I decide which tools are right for me?* We include a wide range of types of tools in this book in order to accommodate a wide range of situations and differences among readers. In our collective sixty-plus years of clinical experience, we've learned that not everyone is the same. Simple idea, but we take this notion very seriously. You may like some of the tools but not others. Some may work for you, while others may not. So, in this chapter, we provide a self-assessment test to identify which types of tools may be better suited to you. But before we do that, let's get a better picture of your current emotional well-being.

HOW ARE YOU FEELING?

First, please get a sharpened pencil with an eraser. In general, it's probably a good idea to have pencils and pens nearby whenever you're reading this book. Since we will be asking you at times to write things down on paper, you should also get a notebook or journal.

To get a better idea of the type of negative emotions that you are currently experiencing, answer the following questions by circling Yes or No. Be as honest as possible. There is no right or wrong answer. This test is to help you better understand your emotions *these days*. Don't spend too much time on any question, but be sure to answer every one.

FEELINGS TEST

Today's date: _____

1. Do you feel sad or down much of the day?   Yes   No

2. Do you feel tired and fatigued, like you have less energy than before?   Yes   No

3. Do you often get upset at people who act as if they are better than you?   Yes   No

4. Do you find yourself yelling at people who wronged you (for example, cut in front of you on the grocery line or honked at you in the car) for several minutes after the event happened?   Yes   No

5. Do you often feel out of breath when you are not exercising?   Yes   No

6. Do you get very angry when you are the butt of a joke?   Yes   No

7. Do you often have feelings of worthlessness or guilt?   Yes   No

8. Do you frequently experience feelings of fear or dread?   Yes   No

9. Do you often have cold feet or hands?   Yes   No

10. Do you often feel hopeless and pessimistic?   Yes   No

11. Do you often say to yourself, *What a jerk this person is?*   Yes   No

12. Do you get angry at people who are rude?   Yes   No

13. Do you have thoughts about harming yourself?   Yes   No

14. Have you lost interest in activities that you used to find pleasurable?   Yes   No

15. Do you frequently feel like your head is about to explode because you get so angry?   Yes   No

16. Do you feel restless or have tight muscles?   Yes   No

17. Do you have problems concentrating or making decisions?   Yes   No

18. Do you get angry frequently?   Yes   No

19. Do you frequently say to yourself, *Why doesn't this person just shut up?*   Yes   No

20. Do you have problems with going to sleep, waking up in the middle of the night, or oversleeping?   Yes   No

21. Do you have headaches, stomachaches, or other pains that are not connected to a medical problem?   Yes   No

22. Have you been rough with people who are annoying to you?   Yes   No

23. Have you lost interest in sex?   Yes   No

24.	Do you sweat or perspire a lot?	Yes	No
25.	Do you often find yourself yelling at someone but forget why you originally got angry?	Yes	No
26.	Do you often have intrusive thoughts about a traumatic event that you experienced?	Yes	No
27.	Do you often get angry at people who violate one of your basic beliefs, values, or principles?	Yes	No
28.	Are you afraid of the future?	Yes	No
29.	Do you often get angry when people are taking too long to do something (for example, taking too long at the post office counter or driving slowly in front of you)?	Yes	No
30.	Do you worry a lot about things in general?	Yes	No
31.	Do you experience dizziness or light-headedness?	Yes	No
32.	Have you lost or gained weight without really trying to?	Yes	No
33.	Do you often feel uncertain and uneasy about what is happening in your life?	Yes	No

Scoring the Feelings Test

Now score the test according to these three feelings: depression, anxiety, and anger.

Depression

Go back and count all of the Yes answers to the following twelve questions: 1, 2, 7, 10, 13, 14, 17, 20, 21, 23, 30, and 32.

Write this number here in pencil: _____

If you answered Yes to fewer than three of these questions, you are probably doing well in general in this area and may not need to read the chapter on depression unless something changes in your life. However, you may simply find chapter 4 interesting reading even if it does not pertain to you directly.

If you answered Yes to three or four of these questions, you are experiencing some of the symptoms of depression currently, but not to a significant extent. You may find it worthwhile to read chapter 4 in order to prevent such symptoms from getting worse.

If you answered Yes to five or more, you should definitely read chapter 4 and follow the directions in that section. The more Yes answers you have among this group of questions, the more likely that you are experiencing depression serious enough to warrant your taking an active role to better manage such feelings.

If you answered Yes to question 13 in particular ("Do you have thoughts about harming yourself?"), you should seriously consider seeking professional advice from a psychologist, counselor, or other medical professional as soon as possible. Perhaps your heart doctor can be of help if you need a referral to a mental-health professional.

Anxiety

Now go back to the test again and count all of the Yes answers to the following twelve questions: 5, 8, 9, 16, 20, 21, 24, 26, 28, 30, 31, and 33.

Write this number here in pencil: _____

If you answered Yes to fewer than three of these questions, you are probably doing well in this area and may not need to read chapter 5 on anxiety unless something changes in your life. However, you may simply find this chapter interesting reading even though it may not pertain to you directly.

If you answered Yes to three or four of these questions, you are currently experiencing some of the symptoms of anxiety, but not to a significant extent. You may find it worthwhile to read chapter 5 in order to prevent such symptoms from getting worse.

If you answered Yes to five or more of these questions, you should definitely read chapter 5 and follow the suggestions in that section. The more Yes answers you have among this group of questions, the more likely that you are experiencing anxiety serious enough that you could benefit from actively addressing it.

Anger

Now go back and count all of the Yes answers to the following twelve questions: 3, 4, 6, 11, 12, 15, 18, 19, 22, 25, 27, and 29.

Write this number here in pencil: _____

If you answered Yes to fewer than three of these questions, you are probably doing well in this area and may not need to read chapter 6 on anger unless something changes in your life. However, you may simply find this chapter interesting reading even though it may not pertain to you directly.

If you answered Yes to three or four of these questions, you are having some difficulty with managing your anger, but not to a significant extent. You may find it worthwhile to read chapter 6 in order to prevent such problems from getting worse.

If you answered Yes to five or more, you should definitely read chapter 6 and follow the advice in that chapter. The more Yes answers you have among this group of questions, the more likely that you are experiencing difficulties with managing feelings of anger and hostility that are serious enough to warrant your taking an active role to better manage such feelings.

What If You Are Directed to More Than One Chapter?

If it turns out that you had four or more Yes answers to two or three of the above sets of questions regarding the three major negative emotions, then you should first go to that chapter for which you have the highest number of Yes answers. You may ultimately find that a particular tool can be helpful in managing symptoms or problems across several areas. But be sure to read those other chapters that are relevant for you as well.

What If You Have Low Scores on All Three Tests?

Remember Karen from the last chapter? She was interested in reducing her emotional distress as a preventive measure. If you were as honest as possible with yourself in answering all the questions and you have low scores on all three subtests, you may wish to read this book simply as a means of fostering overall good health and preventing problems. It's similar to taking aspirin or vitamins or eating healthily to improve your heart health before any problems arise.

The Importance of Being Honest

Shakespeare's words "To thine own self be true" encourage us to be honest with ourselves. Many times people are unaware of how they really feel and how they come across to other people. Take Stan, for example, a sixty-two-year-old man married to Gail for many years. Both sought counseling because Gail felt that they had been having too many problems ever since Stan completed a cardiac rehabilitation program after recovering from a heart attack. During one of the initial counseling sessions, Stan was asked whether he got very angry when he was the butt of a joke. His immediate response was, "I have a great sense of humor. I would never get angry at a good joke!" When Gail was asked if this was true about Stan, she sighed, looked at her husband, and asked him not to get angry at her answer. "Stan does have a good sense of humor. However, he can dish it out but hates getting it back. He may not yell at the time, but he can go on and on in a huff later that night if someone made a joke at his expense. Stan can get real angry! He just doesn't realize it. I don't say anything because I'm afraid if I do, he will only get more angry and that will be bad for his heart."

Because it's hard at times to get a good look at your "inner self," you may be unaware of how you really act, especially if you don't want to admit that you are anxious or feel depressed. It may be a good idea to ask someone close to you for a different perspective. That way, you can get an additional point of view to help you understand how you really feel and come across to others.

At the end of this book is printed the same "Feelings Test" as before, except this one should be completed by someone close to you—your spouse, family member, or close friend. Ask this person to simply answer the questions honestly. Be sure to state very clearly that you won't get upset about the answers. Have this person complete the test privately.

Now use the same scoring instructions and share your answers with each other. Do your best not to get upset if the answers are different. The idea here is for you to have the opportunity to really get to know yourself better by having someone you trust be honest with you. On your own, you might underestimate your difficulties. On the other hand, you might be overly critical of yourself and answer in ways that overestimate your distress. If Gail hadn't been honest with Stan, we would never have been able to help them both manage Stan's anger more effectively. After a few counseling sessions using the tools we'll teach in this book, Stan was able to better understand why he got angry, when he got angry, and—most importantly—how to manage that anger more effectively so it wouldn't damage his relationship with his wife. As a result, he was able to significantly improve his general emotional well-being as part of an overall heart-healthy lifestyle.

After this discussion with your spouse, family member, or friend, go back again and rescore your "Feelings Test" by taking into account any differences in your answers. Be open to the other person's opinions and try hard not to discount them. If your answers are different but you genuinely feel that your answers are more valid than your spouse's or friend's, then don't make any changes. However, do make any changes that appear to be valid. That's why we recommended that you use a pencil (rather than a pen) when you first took this test. The idea is to be as honest with yourself as possible. Your heart is worth it.

Based on the results of your "Feelings Test," check off (in pen this time) your specific goals.

- ☐   decrease depression

- ☐   decrease anxiety

- ☐   manage anger better

You may wish to briefly scan chapter 4 for depression, chapter 5 for anxiety, and chapter 6 for anger at this time. But before you decide which tools to use to meet your goals, you may also wish to determine which self-help strategies may be best suited to your personality. It's time to take another test in the following section.

HOW TO DECIDE WHICH TOOLS ARE BEST FOR YOU

To help you decide which tools are right for you, we will provide specific suggestions about those strategies that are especially helpful for managing depression, anxiety, and anger. In addition, if you are currently seeing a professional (for example, a psychologist or counselor), you may wish to discuss this with him or her for added guidance. Previous success with a given strategy is also a good indicator that a particular tool would be effective once again. For example, you may have learned a particular relaxation tool to help you manage your stress several years ago. If it worked then, it is likely to be helpful now.

However, we do not assume that everybody is the same—in other words, that everybody who experiences depression, for example, does so in the exact same way and for the exact same reasons. Of course, there are many similarities among people who experience the same problem. But there are also differences, especially with regard to what strategies work best for them. Therefore, we have divided the tools into the following seven categories:

- emotional tools

- behavioral action tools

- thinking tools

- relaxation tools

- visualization tools

- interpersonal tools

- spirituality tools

We do not want to pigeonhole anybody by stating that certain people can only be helped by one type of tool. In fact, we believe that the more directions you approach a problem from, the more likely you will be successful in achieving your goals. In other words, for the person experiencing anxiety, an overall plan including thinking tools, visualization tools, and spirituality tools, for example, is more likely to ultimately be successful, as compared to a plan using only one type of tool.

Certain types of tools may be effective for particular people because of individual preferences or differences in symptoms, reactions, or problems. We will provide specific advice in chapters 4, 5, and 6, when we discuss which tools can be particularly helpful to address certain symptoms or reactions regarding depression, anxiety, and anger. This will be one major guide to deciding which tools are suited for you. In addition, you may wish to consider your own individual preferences when making such decisions. To do so, take the following test.

WHICH TOOLS ARE BEST FOR YOU?

Take out your pencil or pen once again and answer the following questions by checking the box that best represents your beliefs. Remember, there are no right or wrong answers. Your answers will help you quickly identify those tools that might be right for you.

1. Are emotional tools right for you?
    In general, do you tend to react emotionally (that is, feel sad, worried, or angry) in response to stressful situations? Do your feelings tend to overshadow your thinking?

    Does this describe you?   ☐ Yes   ☐ No   ☐ Somewhat

    If you answered Yes, it is likely that you will find the tools in chapters 7, 8, 9, and 10 especially suited for you. If you answered Somewhat, you may wish to consider reading these chapters for additional help.

2. Are behavioral action tools right for you?
    Some people are very action-oriented and like to get things done in order to feel a sense of success. When faced with problems, they often want to do something about it to change the situation.

    Does this describe you?   ☐ Yes   ☐ No   ☐ Somewhat

    If you answered Yes, it is likely that you will find the tools in chapter 11 especially suited for you. If you answered Somewhat, you may wish to consider reading chapter 11 for additional help.

3. Are thinking tools right for you?
    Some people have repetitive or troublesome thoughts, images, or memories that trigger negative feelings and distressful moods. They tend to think negative thoughts.

    Does this describe you?   ☐ Yes   ☐ No   ☐ Somewhat

    If you answered Yes, it is likely that you will find the tools in chapters 12 and 13 especially suited for you. If you answered Somewhat, you may wish to consider reading these chapters for additional help.

4. Are relaxation tools right for you?
    Some people experience the world physically. When they are depressed, they get tired and lose their appetite. When they get anxious, their heart beats fast, their palms sweat, and they experience symptoms of panic.

    Does this describe you?   ☐ Yes   ☐ No   ☐ Somewhat

If you answered Yes, it is likely that you will find the tools in chapters 14, 15, and 16 especially suited for you. If you answered Somewhat, you may wish to consider reading these chapters for additional help.

5.   Are visualization tools right for you?
     Some people have the ability to use their "mind's eye." When they think of things, they tend to be able to see them in their mind. It is like thinking in pictures. Such people like to use their imagination and visualize things.

     Does this describe you?   ☐ Yes   ☐ No   ☐ Somewhat

If you answered Yes, it is likely that you will find the tools in chapters 17 and 18 especially suited for you. If you answered Somewhat, you may wish to consider reading these chapters for additional help.

6.   Are interpersonal tools right for you?
     Some people like working with other people or feel that friends are very important to them. Not having support from friends and family members makes them feel sad and upset.

     Does this describe you?   ☐ Yes   ☐ No   ☐ Somewhat

If you answered Yes, it is likely that you will find the tools in chapter 19 especially suited to you. If you answered Somewhat, you may wish to consider reading this chapter for additional help.

7.   Are spirituality tools right for you?
     Some people think of a higher power as being a core part of their life. This higher power could be God, Jesus, or Allah—in terms of a formal religion—or could be a belief in the universality of the world. When thinking about their life, their future, and their happiness, such people tend to couch such thoughts within a spiritual or faith-based framework.

     Does this describe you?   ☐ Yes   ☐ No   ☐ Somewhat

If you answered Yes, it is likely that you will find the tools in chapter 20 especially suited for you. If you answered Somewhat, you may wish to consider reading this chapter for additional help.

What Is Your Tool Chest Profile?

Go back over the above test and indicate below those categories of strategies that appear to be suited for you in particular (that is, any category where you answered yes) by checking them off under the A column. These are the tools you are most likely to find helpful. Not that the others tools won't help—rather, think of this as your A-list of tools.

Tools	A	B
emotional tools	☐	☐
behavioral action tools	☐	☐
thinking tools	☐	☐
relaxation tools	☐	☐
visualization tools	☐	☐
interpersonal tools	☐	☐
spirituality tools	☐	☐

Now go back over your answers to the above questions once again and check off those categories of strategies for which you answered somewhat, this time under the B column. These tools are likely to be helpful as well. Think of these, in part, as your plan B in case those on the A-list are not helping sufficiently.

The old saying "Many roads lead to Rome" suggests that there are many ways to reach your goal, and we believe that different "roads" may be good for different people. A good tool for one person may not be a good tool for another. That's why you should try many different tools. Eventually, you will be able to pick and choose those that are right for you. We believe that many of the tools, even those in the categories that you did not rate highly, can be of help.

When trying to choose the tools that are best suited for you, remember that "the more arrows you shoot, the more likely you will hit the target." In other words, the more tools you use, the more likely it is that you will succeed in achieving your goals.

ADDITIONAL ADVICE AND HINTS

Beyond the tools themselves, we believe there are important ideas to consider in how you go about using the tools. These include

- how you read this book,

- how often you use the tools,

- how you note when things are not getting better (or are getting worse) in order to determine when you should shift gears and choose another tool to use, and

- how you react when things are getting better.

Read Actively, Not Passively

Having already been directed to take tests and get pencils, pens, and notepads, you realize that this book is asking you to be interactive rather than to simply read the text. We firmly believe that you will get a lot more out of this book if you take an active role in using it. What does this mean? When you read the newspaper or a novel, you probably tend to be more passive in the way you approach the material. That's fine, especially if you're reading a novel, for example, for your pleasure. However, with a self-help book such as this one, it is best to be more active. Read more slowly, stop when you have a question, and take the time to really think about what is being said. Don't skip over parts of a chapter in order to see how it ends. Think about different situations in your life where a particular tool could be useful. Think about how you might need to change the strategy slightly to adapt to a different situation. Think about how you might share your experiences with your spouse, friends, or family members. Finally, it is likely that the more you reread sections that are relevant to you, the more you will learn and ultimately be able to change.

Be Persistent and Practice

You might be wondering, *How long should it take before I get better?* This is a legitimate question. If taking the suggestions in this book seriously does not lead to some change in your life within a three- to six-month period, then maybe it isn't for you. However, when we suggest that you need to take the guidance seriously, that means you need to be persistent and practice the tools according to our suggestions. Think of most of these tools as skills that you are learning for the first time, similar to learning to drive a car or learning a new sport or hobby. Take, for example, learning how to play tennis. It would be silly to think that all you needed to do was read a book quickly and practice only occasionally. If you truly wanted to become a decent tennis player, it is likely that you would want to practice as many times as possible. Sometimes it is a matter of practicing your backhand swing over and over again, and sometimes it involves playing entire matches with someone slightly better than you.

It is in this context that we would like you to understand the process of learning the strategies in this book. For any of the tools to work, you need to practice it more frequently in the beginning. Doing twenty-five sit-ups the first day will not give you a six-pack set of abs that day. Rather, it is the beginning of a journey during which you need to practice in order to succeed. We know that at times it becomes very difficult to persist, especially when progress is slow. However, if your initial attitude is one of accepting that changing your life will take practice and persistence, rather than hoping that this is the magic pill, it is more likely that you will ultimately be successful. Remember, this is for you, and you are worth it. Change takes time. Rome wasn't built in a day, and neither can you expect yourself to change overnight.

Track Your Progress

Would you ever continue writing checks to pay bills or purchase clothes and groceries without attempting to note each amount and keep track of the balance in your account? Of course not! Not keeping track of your progress in learning to manage your emotions would result in a similar problem: you would have little idea what exactly was going on. For many of the tools in this book, we suggest a means of tracking your progress—for example, whether using a particular relaxation tool actually leads to a decrease in feelings of stress. That way, you can determine if your progress is on track or whether you need to use additional tools to reach your goals.

Keeping track of your overall emotional well-being is also important. To do that, simply retake the "Feelings Test" at intervals that are meaningful for you (for example, every four weeks). One way to keep good records is to use your notebook or journal. Simply write the numbers 1 through 33 and answer each of the questions once again, trying to be as honest as possible. Note the date. Go back to the last time you took this test and compare your scores. Is there any progress? How much progress? If you are unsatisfied, take this as a signal that you may need to learn tools that you haven't tried before. In addition, ask yourself whether you have been practicing enough. Take the time to determine a new strategy or plan in using this book. Reread some of the key chapters, and continue to be persistent!

Reward Yourself

Too often, we have heard people who have been successful in improving their emotional well-being say that the change is reward enough in and of itself. We feel differently, and the scientific literature backs us up on this notion (Rehm and Adams 2003). First, we strongly suggest that you reinforce or reward yourself for trying to use a tool. Also, you should reward yourself for making progress. Small changes are very important. Don't wait until you meet your ultimate goal. A big victory is usually made up of a series of smaller ones.

You can reward yourself by buying a new CD, going to the movies, getting tickets to a sports event, buying a new outfit, going to a fancy restaurant, or doing something else that pleases you. Make the reward equal to the progress—for a big success, give yourself a big reward! Make sure that you associate the reward with your effort and progress.

3

Your Heart:
A Primer

In this chapter, we'll talk about your heart and how it works. We'll discuss the major types of heart disease as well as risk factors and treatment options.

The heart is a muscular pump that is about the size of your fist and generally weighs about three-quarters of a pound. It is located to the left of the center of your chest, between your lungs, with the tip (or *apex*) pointing down and to the left. Your spinal column is in back of the heart, and your breastbone or *sternum* helps to protect it from the front. On average, the normal adult heart pumps about 2,000 gallons of blood throughout the body and beats (that is, expands and contracts) about 100,000 times daily.

The heart is the main part of the body's overall circulatory or cardiovascular system. There are approximately 60,000 miles of blood vessels in this system, which includes a network of elastic tubes that carry blood that the heart pumps throughout the other parts of the body. The circulatory system includes the heart, lungs, *arteries* (vessels that carry blood from the heart to various parts of the body), *arterioles* (small branches of arteries), and *capillaries* (very small blood vessels). These types of blood vessels carry oxygen- and nutrient-rich blood throughout the body. In addition, the circulatory system includes veins and *venules* (small veins). These types of blood vessels carry oxygen- and nutrient-depleted blood back to the heart and lungs.

HOW YOUR HEART WORKS

The heart is made up of four chambers through which the blood is pumped. The upper two chambers are the right and left *atria,* while the lower two are the right and left *ventricles.* Your heart works as a pump when it squeezes blood out of its chambers (which is a *contraction*) and then expands to allow blood back in (which is called *relaxation*). The next time you are washing dishes and have a soft plastic bottle, hold it underwater. First squeeze water out of the bottle and then release your grasp. Note how water is sucked back into the bottle. This is essentially how your heart works.

You can think of the ventricles as the pumping room and the atria as the receiving rooms. The chambers work together in an organized sequence of contractions. First, an electrical signal starts the heartbeat by causing the atria to contract, which allows the relaxed ventricles to fill up with blood. Next, the ventricles discharge blood as the atria now relax and become filled up. The right side of your heart pumps blood to your lungs, where it receives oxygen and gets rid of carbon dioxide. The left side receives this oxygen-rich blood from the lungs and then pumps it to the tissues and other organs of your body. The "used" blood ("used" because it has already delivered oxygen and nutrients to the tissues) returning from the tissues has to circulate through the lungs before it enters the left chambers. This blood is a dark bluish red because it is oxygen-depleted. When the blood goes through the lungs to receive oxygen once again, it becomes bright red.

Among other organs of the body (such as the stomach and intestines), the muscles of the heart are regulated by the *autonomic nervous system* (ANS), which is part of the body's overall peripheral nervous system. The ANS works in a reflexive and involuntary manner, helping your body to react appropriately to various situations. In particular, the ANS is important in how you react to two different types of situations. In the first circumstance, which involves a stressful or scary situation (for example, if you are confronted by a lion, an angry boss, or a stolen car), the *sympathetic nervous system,* a part of the ANS, is called into action by using your body's energy to help you either "fight the lion" or "run away from it." Automatically, in preparing your body to do either task, this part of the ANS increases your blood pressure, increases your heart rate, and slows down your digestion, among other activities. In the second situation, which involves nonemergencies and restful circumstances, the *parasympathetic nervous system,* another part of the ANS, is called into play. This system is responsible for helping your body to save energy. When you are resting, this system automatically decreases your blood pressure, decreases your heart rate, and allows digestion to begin, among other activities.

YOUR BLOOD PRESSURE

In general, it takes more pressure to circulate blood throughout the body as compared to circulating it through the lungs. Therefore, it stands to reason that the left side of your heart is stronger than the right side, because it needs to generate more pressure. Blood pressure is a measurement of the pressure in your blood vessels throughout the body. It should be measured when you are resting quietly. Your physician uses a *sphygmomanometer,* which consists of a cuff and a gauge, to take your blood pressure. The cuff goes around your arm, and the gauge, which looks like a thermometer, contains mercury. The scientific abbreviation for mercury is Hg. This is why a blood pressure reading is conveyed in terms of millimeters (mm) of mercury (Hg). For example, an average blood pressure might be presented as 120 mm Hg over 70 mm Hg.

The top number (that is, 120 mm Hg in this example) represents the *systolic* blood pressure. This is the pressure in the arteries of your arm when your heart is squeezing blood out into your circulatory system. The bottom number (that is, 70 mm Hg) is the *diastolic* blood pressure and represents the pressure in the arteries of your arm when your heart relaxes between beats.

High Blood Pressure

High blood pressure, or *hypertension,* occurs when a person's blood pressure is consistently above a normal range. In an adult, high blood pressure is defined as a consistent systolic pressure of 140 mm Hg or higher and/or a diastolic pressure of 90 mm Hg or higher. Blood pressure of less than 120 over 80 mm Hg is generally considered normal for adults.

High blood pressure is potentially harmful because it causes the heart to work harder than normal. In addition, high blood pressure can lead to increased risk for heart attacks, strokes, kidney failure, arteriosclerosis ("hardening" of the arteries), and other physical problems. In about 90 to 95 percent of all cases, the cause of hypertension is unknown. The medical term for this type of high blood pressure is *essential hypertension. Secondary hypertension* describes those cases where the cause is known (for example, kidney abnormality or birth defect of parts of the arterial system).

HEART RATE

Your *heart rate* refers to the number of beats per minute your heart makes. In normal resting adults, the heart rate is generally between sixty and one hundred beats per minute. With increased activity, such as running, climbing stairs, or exercising, your heart rate speeds up in order to pump more blood to your muscles. As you get older, your heart rate begins to slow down. Also, your heart rate can become slower with improved physical conditioning; for example, an athlete's heart tends to be stronger and actually pumps more blood with each contraction. Thus the athlete's heart is not required to beat as fast in order to have a normal blood flow.

HEART DISEASE

There are many different types of heart disease, and they vary in seriousness, impact, and overt symptoms. Collectively, cardiovascular diseases are the number one killer in the United States of both men and women. Although people still tend to believe that heart disease is a man's disease, the statistics tell a different story. For example, according to the American Heart Association (2004), heart disease causes approximately one death per minute among women, claiming nearly half a million female lives per year in the United States. Further, beginning at age seventy-five, the *prevalence* (that is, an estimate of how many people have a specific disease at a given time) of heart disease is higher among women than among men.

In 2001, about sixty-four million Americans (or 22.6 percent of the overall population) had one or more forms of heart disease. Approximately half of these individuals (thirty-one million) were men and half (thirty-three million) were women. Heart disease accounted for close to 44 percent of all deaths in the United States in 2001 (approximately one of every 2.6 deaths). Heart disease not only has a devastating effect on health and well-being, it also exacts a huge financial cost. For example, in 2004, the estimated direct and indirect cost of heart disease was $368.4 billion (American Heart Association 2004).

In this section, we provide a brief overview of the major forms of heart disease.

Coronary Heart Disease

Ischemia refers to the condition where the flow of blood to a part of the body is restricted. *Cardiac ischemia* represents a lack of blood flow and oxygen to the heart. *Coronary heart disease* (CHD), also called *coronary artery disease* and *ischemic heart disease,* refers to problems caused by arteries that are clogged or narrowed. When the arteries are narrow, it becomes more difficult for blood and oxygen to reach the heart. CHD can lead to a heart attack. Ischemia can often cause chest pain or discomfort. The medical term for chest pain is *angina.*

Arteries can become narrow as a result of *atherosclerosis,* a form of arteriosclerosis, which is a process that begins in childhood and progresses as people get older. This disease involves deposits of fatty substances, calcium, cholesterol, and other substances that build up on the inner lining of an artery. This buildup is referred to as *plaque* and generally occurs on large and medium-sized arteries.

It is generally believed that atherosclerosis progresses when the inner layer of the artery, the *endothelium,* is damaged. Three known causes of such damage are

- heightened levels of *cholesterol* (a fatlike substance that is produced by the liver) and *triglyceride* (the most common type of fat in the body),

- high blood pressure, and

- tobacco smoke.

As a result of damage to the endothelium, various substances—such as *platelets* (a blood element that helps in blood clotting), fats, and cholesterol—become deposited in the artery wall and can build up and form plaque. When this plaque becomes large enough to thicken the artery wall, the diameter of the artery shrinks, significantly reducing blood flow and the critical oxygen supply to the heart.

Heart Attack

The medical term for a heart attack is *myocardial infarction,* or MI. Heart attacks are caused by coronary heart disease as a function of stoppage or significant reduction of the blood supply to the heart. This blood flow becomes reduced as a result of atherosclerosis. Sometimes the plaque buildup in an artery ruptures, causing a blood clot or *thrombus* to form and totally block blood flow in the artery. When such a blood clot blocks a blood vessel that supplies the heart, a heart attack can occur. The medical term for this type of heart attack is *coronary thrombosis.*

If the blood supply to the heart is cut off for more than a few minutes, muscle cells can be permanently damaged. An *infarct* is the area of tissue that has been damaged due to the lack of oxygen and other nutrients usually supplied by the blood. If no clot has occurred, a heart attack can occur if the artery is significantly blocked for longer than thirty minutes to two hours. Although heart attacks are often associated with severe anginal pain, it is also possible to have a "silent" heart attack (called *silent ischemia*), where there are no overt symptoms. The American Heart Association (2004) notes that as many as three to four million Americans have such episodes each year without knowing it.

A heart attack can lead to immediate death because of extensive damage to the heart. If the damage is minor and the heart's electrical system is not greatly affected, chances are good that the person will survive the heart attack. Unfortunately, any heart attack can lead to further complications or heart problems. For example, if 25 percent or more of the heart is damaged, it may become enlarged, and *heart failure* (the group of diseases where the heart is unable to adequately circulate enough blood throughout the body) can develop. In addition, if the pumping function of the left ventricle is damaged, various disturbances of the heart's rhythms can occur.

Symptoms of a heart attack include the following:

- intense chest pain or feelings of heavy pressure

- pain that starts from the chest and radiates to the left shoulder and arm

- continuous pain in the upper abdomen

- shortness of breath

- fainting

- nausea, vomiting, and sweating

As with men, the most common heart attack symptom for women is chest pain or discomfort. However, women are more likely than men to have other warning signs, particularly shortness of breath, nausea, vomiting, and back or jaw pain.

Arrhythmias

Arrhythmias, also called *dysrhythmias*, are abnormal heart rhythms. These can cause the heart to work less effectively. Remember that the heart has four chambers, the top two being the atria and the bottom two being the ventricles. The heart's own natural pacemaker is a group of cells called the *sinoatrial* (or SA) *node*, which is located on the top of the right atrium. The SA node is important to the heart because it sends an initial electrical signal throughout the atria that begins the heartbeat. This electrical signal reaches a second node, the *atrioventricular* (or AV) *node*, which is located toward the top of the left ventricle. The signal continues to travel from the AV node through a group of fibers in the ventricle and eventually spreads to all parts of both ventricles. Think of the SA and AV nodes as being responsible for your normal heart rate and rhythm. Without the electrical signal following this route, the heart would not function properly.

An arrhythmia, then, represents a change from this normal sequence of electrical signals and impulses. Many arrhythmias are brief and have little effect on a person's heart rate. However, if the arrhythmias exist for a time, they can change the overall heart rate, making it too fast, too slow, or erratic. The medical term for an abnormally slow heart rate is *bradycardia* (that is, a heart rate of fewer than sixty beats per minute), while the term for a heart rate that is too fast is *tachycardia* (that is, a heart rate of greater than one hundred beats per minute).

In general, the symptoms and consequences of arrhythmias are broad in scope, ranging from no perceptible symptoms to cardiac arrest and sudden cardiac death. Tachycardia (also termed *tachyarrhythmia*) involves rapid heart beating, which can reduce the heart's effectiveness in pumping and circulating blood. This can lead to palpitations ("skipped" heartbeats), dizziness, light-headedness, and fainting. Rapid heart beating that begins in the ventricles (*ventricular tachycardia*) can lead to ventricular *fibrillation* (fast, uncoordinated contractions), where the heart becomes unable to function as a pump. This disorder can lead to death or cause serious damage to other organs.

Bradycardia can also lead to clinical symptoms. Because the heart may not be able to pump sufficient blood throughout the body, bradycardia can cause fatigue, light-headedness, and fainting.

Cardiomyopathy

Cardiomyopathy is the disease where the heart muscle itself becomes significantly less effective as a pump. There are three types of cardiomyopathy—dilated, hypertrophic, and restrictive.

Dilated or *congestive* cardiomyopathy is the most common form and occurs when the heart cavity is enlarged and stretched. The heart becomes weak and loses its ability to pump blood effectively. Often, *congestive heart failure* (the condition where the heart cannot pump enough blood to other organs in the body) results. Symptoms can include shortness of breath and *edema* (swelling).

Hypertrophic cardiomyopathy involves the enlargement and thickening (or *hypertrophy*) of the muscle mass of the left ventricle. This blocks blood flow and can lead to arrhythmias and abnormal heartbeats. Symptoms can include shortness of breath, dizziness, fainting, and chest pain.

The least common form of this disease, *restrictive cardiomyopathy*, occurs when the *myocardium* (the muscle wall) of the ventricles becomes excessively rigid. It becomes more difficult for the ventricles to fill up with blood between heartbeats. People with this disease may feel tired, have swollen hands and feet, and have difficulty breathing upon exertion.

RISK FACTORS FOR HEART DISEASE

A *risk factor* is a trait or lifestyle habit that increases the statistical likelihood that a person will experience a disease. The more risk factors you have, the more likely it is that you will experience heart disease. Some risk factors for coronary heart disease and heart attacks are controllable, while others are not. For example, risk factors that cannot be changed include increasing age, male gender, race (African Americans have a greater chance of having high blood pressure and a higher risk for heart disease compared to Caucasians), and family history.

The following risk factors can be controlled through medical treatment or lifestyle changes:

- high blood pressure

- diabetes

- smoking tobacco

- high blood cholesterol

- physical inactivity

- obesity

- excessive alcohol consumption

- stress and negative emotions

The major purpose of this book is to underscore how negative emotions, specifically depression, anxiety, and anger, serve as potential risk factors for heart disease. By controlling these risk factors, you can reduce your risk of heart disease.

TREATMENT OPTIONS

Treatment options for heart diseases include medication, surgery, and lifestyle changes.

Medications

Numerous medications are available to treat various heart problems and related symptoms. For example, high blood pressure is treated with *antihypertensives*, such as *diuretics* (which reduce excess fluids and salt), *angiotensin converting enzyme* (ACE) *inhibitors* (which interfere with the body's production of a chemical that causes arterioles to constrict), and *beta blockers* (which block the ability of the sympathetic nervous system to constrict blood vessels). Another class of drugs, called *vasodilators*, help blood vessels to dilate or widen.

For people who have experienced a heart attack, *nitroglycerin* is a commonly prescribed medication. This drug helps to relax the veins and coronary arteries in order to increase the heart's blood supply. In addition, a variety of antiarrhthymic drugs are used to treat tachycardias and premature heartbeats.

Medications, such as aspirin, that reduce the "stickiness" of platelets (called *antiplatelet agents*) and thus help to reduce the ability of the blood to coagulate are also commonly used in patients with heart disease. Further, a variety of medications are routinely prescribed to help individuals lower their cholesterol levels.

Surgery

Various surgical procedures are used to treat a variety of heart problems. For example, *balloon angioplasty* (also known as *percutaneous transluminal coronary angioplasty* or PTCA), is a procedure used to widen narrowed coronary arteries. The cardiologist uses a catheter with a balloon at its tip to open up a blockage in an artery by compressing the plaque and stretching the artery open. A more recent advancement in this type of technology is the *coronary stent*. A stent is a wire mesh tube that is used to prop open an artery that has recently been dilated and cleared via angioplasty. When the balloon is inflated, the stent expands to form a scaffold and remains in place permanently in order to improve blood flow and reduce chest pain.

Another type of surgical procedure involves bypassing certain clogged arteries in order to improve the supply of oxygen-rich blood to the heart. Often referred to as a "cabbage" (that is, CABG, for *coronary artery bypass graft*), this surgery takes a blood vessel from another part of the body in order to make a detour around the blocked part of the artery. Blood can then flow freely in this new channel.

Medical procedures involving surgical implantation of certain devices are also used to treat arrhythmias. For example, a *pacemaker* can be inserted on the left side of the heart, under the skin below the collarbone, in order to treat life-threatening bradycardia. This device consists of a pulse generator the size of a silver dollar.

Pacemakers deliver electrical signals to the heart when the spontaneous heart rate falls below a set value.

Similarly, the *implantable cardioverter defibrillator*, or ICD, is implanted in order to treat *sustained ventricular tachycardia* (abnormally fast heart rate). This device, generally implanted under the skin just below the collarbone, senses the heart's rhythms and paces the heart when necessary. When it detects ventricular tachycardia, the ICD actually delivers a shock to the heart in order to restore it to a normal rhythm. Newer versions can also serve as a pacemaker if bradycardia occurs. ICDs have been found to be especially effective in reducing sudden cardiac death that results from ventricular tachycardia.

Lifestyle Changes

A significant part of a comprehensive treatment plan for existing heart disease is overcoming any and all risk factors that can be controlled. For example, if you have already experienced a heart attack and you're obese, you smoke, and you deal with stress ineffectively, your treatment plan should include ameliorating these influences. Many of the risk factors noted previously involve changing behavior in order to, for example, reduce weight, improve diet, increase exercise, stop smoking tobacco, and improve your ability to manage stress. While there are several medical treatments that are potentially effective for changing such behaviors (for example, the nicotine patch to decrease cigarette smoking), psychological interventions are very effective means to change lifestyle habits. We have written this self-help guide with a specific focus on overcoming negative emotions in order to improve your heart health.

Part 2

Understanding
Your Emotions

4

Depression and Heart Disease

Depression usually involves sustained feelings of sadness or loss of interest in activities that were previously enjoyed. It is a very common disorder, occurring in as many as one in four people. It's called a disorder because, like many illnesses, it is diagnosed based on the presence of a group of upsetting symptoms that don't go away after a few days. Because of its high prevalence among the general population, it is often referred to as the "common cold" of emotional disorders.

Depression is also relatively common among heart patients. For example, it has been reported to be as high as 45 percent among post–heart attack patients and 40 percent among patients with ischemic heart disease (Jiang et al. 2002). Depression among heart patients tends to be underdiagnosed, which is extremely unfortunate because depression has been shown to be associated with high rates of further cardiac complications (for example, death or another heart attack) as well as with poor adherence to cardiac rehabilitation and medical treatment. Being depressed has also been found to actually increase medical costs by 40 percent for heart patients experiencing such symptoms, as compared to heart patients not experiencing depression (Frasure-Smith et al. 2000).

SYMPTOMS OF DEPRESSION

The following are symptoms of depression:

- ☐ feelings of sadness

- ☐ significant decrease or loss of interest in activities that used to be pleasurable

- ☐ lack of energy, fatigue, feelings of being "slowed down"

- ☐ feelings of emptiness and anxiety

- ☐ problems with sleep (having difficulty falling asleep, waking up early in the morning, or oversleeping)

- ☐ changes in appetite or actual weight (increase or decrease that is not deliberately planned)

- ☐ recurrent thoughts of suicide and death, suicide attempts

- ☐ feelings of pessimism and hopelessness

- ☐ feelings of worthlessness and guilt

- ☐ difficulties in concentrating and making decisions and problems with memory

- ☐ minor physical symptoms (headaches, stomachaches) not caused by physical illness

You don't have to have all of these symptoms to be depressed. In general, significant depression means having about five of the above symptoms, one of which involves feelings of sadness or a decrease in pleasure or interest in most activities. What are your symptoms? Get a pen or pencil and go back over this list of symptoms, checking off those that are particularly troubling to you. This will be helpful later in this chapter when we provide guidance as to which tools may be helpful for your particular symptoms of depression.

Your scores in the depression section of the "Feelings Test" in chapter 1 (questions 1, 2, 7, 10, 13, 14, 17, 20, 21, 23, 30, and 32) can serve as a baseline against which you can measure your progress as you use self-help strategies. In other words, that particular score (that is, the number of questions to which you answered Yes) offers an indication of how you are currently doing. Retaking this section of the "Feelings Test" after about a month of applying certain tools can be an easy way to measure your progress, just like using a thermometer to check your temperature.

DEPRESSION AND HEART DISEASE

Depression has been found to be an important risk factor for heart disease. Specifically, depression is significantly linked to the initial development of heart problems, and it increases your risk for further complications and potentially lethal problems if you are already experiencing some type of heart disease (Thomas et al. 2003).

Depression as a Risk Factor for Initial Heart Disease

As we've said, this type of negative emotion or feeling is fairly common among heart patients. Obviously, feeling depressed leads to a poor quality of life. However, research has demonstrated that depression can increase the risk for heart disease even in disease-free individuals. For example, following a group of 1,190 male medical students over a period of forty years, researchers at the Johns Hopkins University School of Medicine found that depressed men were at a significantly greater risk (twofold, or 200 percent) for developing both coronary heart disease and myocardial infarction compared to individuals who were not depressed (Ford et al. 1998).

In addition, Barefoot and Schroll (1996) evaluated the role of depression in the initial development of coronary disease among 409 men and 321 women, all of whom were born in the same year (1914) in Glostrup, Denmark. These researchers found that high levels of depressive symptoms were associated with increased risks of both initial myocardial infarctions and cardiac-related death, even after controlling for other risk factors (for example, smoking, high blood pressure, and decreased physical activity) and signs of disease at the baseline evaluation. In addition, they noted that men and women were equally vulnerable to heart disease if they were depressed.

In a prospective study entitled the National Health Examination Follow-Up Study, among a group of 2,832 healthy adults, depression was found to be associated with a significant increased risk of both fatal and nonfatal ischemic heart disease (Anda et al. 1993).

Last, in a recent quantitative review of studies that assessed the association between depression and coronary heart disease, researchers concluded that depressive symptoms represent a significant independent risk for the onset of coronary disease (Wulsin and Singal 2003). Although these researchers suggest that such a risk is less than that related to active smoking, they conclude that depression involves a greater risk for an initial coronary problem than that presented by secondhand smoke.

Depression and the Risk of Further Heart Problems and Death

Depression among patients with various types of heart disease also increases the risk of additional heart problems and even death. For example, researchers in Montreal, Canada, followed a group of 896 individuals aged twenty-four to eighty-eight for a period of five years following a heart attack. They found that negative mood and depression significantly predicted cardiac-related deaths independent of the severity of heart disease (Frasure-Smith and Lespérance 2003).

Further, among a sample of 438 Japanese heart patients, experiencing depression after an acute myocardial infarction was found to be a significant predictor of further cardiac events one year after the heart attack, especially among elderly patients (Shiotani et al. 2002).

In a seminal research study that followed a group of 222 patients six months after a heart attack, Frasure-Smith, Lespérance, and Talajic (1993) found that depression was associated with more than a 400 percent increase in the risk of cardiac-related death after adjusting for other risk factors, such as left ventricular dysfunction and previous heart attacks.

In a recent review of the literature investigating the relationship of depression and mortality among patients with heart failure, Thomas and colleagues (2003) concluded that a higher percentage of such patients who were depressed died, compared to those individuals who were not depressed. The relationship between depression and risk for mortality among heart failure patients appears to be *linear;* that is, the greater the level of depression, the higher the risk for cardiac-related death. For example, Vaccarino and colleagues (2001) found that at a six-month follow-up evaluation, mortality rates of depressed individuals were significantly higher than among nondepressed patients. In addition, moderately and severely depressed patients with heart failure had significantly higher death rates than mildly depressed patients with heart failure.

As we mentioned in chapter 3, the implantable cardioverter defibrillator is the treatment of choice for people with sustained ventricular tachycardia or fibrillation (that is, a heart rate of greater than one hundred beats per minute at rest). The ICD shocks the heart in order to restore a normal rhythm only when it detects the fibrillation. That means that an ICD shock is the result of the heart experiencing a life-threatening tachycardia. Research has found that depression increases the likelihood of an ICD discharge or shock, suggesting that depression leads to dangerous arrhythmic activity. For example, Heller and colleagues (1998) found that despite improvement in actual physical health, ICD patients who experienced depression and worried about their health also experienced a higher rate of subsequent ICD shocks. In addition, Dunbar and colleagues (1999) reported that depression that was identified three months after implantation of the ICD predicted subsequent ICD shocks three months later, regardless of the severity of disease and the use of medications.

How Does Depression Lead to Heart Disease?

In chapter 1, we provided some examples of how a negative feeling, such as depression, can have a biological impact on the heart. For those of you who are particularly interested in this topic, we'll further describe various hypotheses that physicians and scientists have suggested as to how this actually works. The explanations we provide in this section represent possible *mechanisms of action,* or reasons why depression can increase the risk for heart disease.

First, depression can lead to poor health in general and may increase the likelihood that a person will engage in risky lifestyles such as overeating, smoking, and lack of exercise. Depression can also decrease a person's willingness and ability to adhere to medical treatment prescriptions. For example, Carney and colleagues (1995) found that during the first few weeks after a *coronary angiography* (a test involving injecting liquid into your arteries in order to determine how well they are working), depressed individuals did not adhere to a prescribed aspirin regimen as well as nondepressed patients.

Depression can also lead to dysregulation of the hypothalamic-pituitary-adrenocortical (HPA) axis. The *HPA axis* is that part of the body's system that coordinates various behavioral, neuroendocrine, autonomic, and immune responses to alterations in homeostasis. *Homeostasis* is the body's ability to maintain the stability of its internal environment, including the cardiovascular system, within certain limits that allow it to survive. In essence, the HPA axis becomes activated when you react to stress, and it affects the immune system. Scientists have suggested that in this manner, depression leads to problems with the body's ability to biologically handle life stress effectively via the HPA axis (Musselman, Evans, and Nemeroff 1998).

Depression has also been found to be strongly linked to reduced heart rate variability (HRV). Greater HRV is associated with good cardiovascular health, because the variability serves to buffer the negative effects of stress on the cardiovascular system. On the other hand, reduced HRV is a known risk factor for sudden cardiac death (Gorman and Sloan 2000).

Last, research has suggested that depression can contribute to heart disease by causing injuries to the endothelium, which is the innermost layer of an artery. When an artery is damaged, platelets hurry to the site of the damage in an effort to stop any bleeding. Depression has also been linked to *smooth muscle proliferation*, which is an increase in smooth muscle cells that are involved in the constriction and dilation of blood vessels. Smooth muscle cell proliferation contributes to the production of plaque in the arteries and the deposit of *lipids* (fatty substances insoluble in blood) at the site of the endothelium damage. Collectively and over time, these processes can lead to atherosclerosis, which can significantly reduce blood flow to the heart (Carney et al. 2002; Musselman et al. 1996).

DEPRESSION CAN BE EFFECTIVELY TREATED

Can depression be effectively treated? The answer is a resounding yes. Both antidepressant medication and certain forms of psychotherapy and counseling have been found to be highly effective in treating depression. The types of psychological treatment approaches that have been shown to be especially effective are under the general umbrella of interventions called *cognitive behavioral therapy*. These include, for example, cognitive therapy, behavioral activation, problem-solving therapy, and self-control therapy. These therapies are scientifically supported, which means that they have been shown to be effective with many depressed patients (Nezu, Nezu, and Lombardo 2004).

The tools we offer in this book are based on these forms of scientifically supported psychotherapies.

WHAT YOU CAN DO NOW ABOUT YOUR DEPRESSION

You can use the self-help strategies contained in this book to help manage your depressive symptoms. To help you decide which tools to use to reduce your depression, we offer the following two guidelines. First, use those types of tools that seem to suit you best, as you determined in the "What Is Your Tool Chest Profile?" exercise in chapter 2. You can go now to the categories of tools on your A-list. Second, use those types of tools that match a particular symptom you are experiencing, even if the tool category is not on your A-list. Use the table below as a guide. This list contains the various symptoms of depression. Go back to the symptom list provided earlier in this chapter and note those symptoms that you checked off as being particularly troubling for you. Find those symptoms on the list below and note which specific strategies are suggested as being particularly useful for each symptom. If you are experiencing symptoms related to appetite changes, fatigue, or difficulties concentrating (they are not specifically noted on the list below), go to the tools associated with symptoms of sad feelings and loss of interest in pleasurable activities.

Symptom	Related Tools
feelings of sadness	"Using Feelings to Better Know Yourself" (chapter 7) "Expressing Emotions Constructively" (chapter 8) "Fostering Acceptance" (chapter 9) "Getting Social Support" (chapter 19) "Awakening Your Spirituality" (chapter 20)
loss of interest in pleasurable activities	"Enhancing Positive Experiences" (chapter 11) "Solving Stressful Problems" (chapter 13)
feelings of anxiety	"Using Feelings to Better Know Yourself" (chapter 7) "Expressing Emotions Constructively" (chapter 8) "Deep Breathing" (chapter 14) "Autogenic Training" (chapter 15) "Deep Muscle Relaxation" (chapter 16) "Mind Travel to a Safe Place" (chapter 17)

sleep difficulties	"Autogenic Training" (chapter 15)
	"Deep Muscle Relaxation" (chapter 16)
feelings of worthlessness, guilt, or hopelessness	"Changing Negative Thinking" (chapter 12)
	"Visualizing Success" (chapter 18)
difficulties making decisions	"Solving Stressful Problems" (chapter 13)
thoughts of suicide	"Enhancing Positive Experiences" (chapter 11)
	"Solving Stressful Problems" (chapter 13)
	"Visualizing Success" (chapter 18)
minor physical symptoms	"Deep Breathing" (chapter 14)
	"Autogenic Training" (chapter 15)
	"Deep Muscle Relaxation" (chapter 16)

YOUR PERSONAL PLAN FOR DEPRESSION

Take out your pen or pencil once again and write down in your notebook or journal your personal plan to help reduce your depression. To begin with, write down at least three tools that you have decided to try as part of an initial overall plan. Make a commitment to learn them and use them to the best of your ability. Remember that as with other skills, like driving a car or playing a sport, you'll need to practice over time in order to get better. Don't get discouraged!

Add tools to this list if necessary. Don't forget that the more arrows you shoot, the more likely you will hit the target. Remember to be an active reader, be persistent and practice applying each tool, track your progress, and reward yourself.

5

Anxiety and Heart Disease

Anxiety is a very common human experience. However, it can become a serious problem when it interferes with your daily activities. Currently, there are over nineteen million Americans suffering from an anxiety disorder (National Institute of Mental Health 2004). Anxiety disorders are the most prevalent type of psychological problem in the United States. There are several different types of anxiety disorders, but in general, anxiety can be thought of as a negative emotion characterized by fear and associated with feelings of worry, apprehension about the future, and a sense of lack of control over events. It is also characterized by various physical symptoms, such as increased heart rate and sweating.

Unfortunately, anxiety tends to be very prevalent among heart patients. For example, Crowne and colleagues (1996) found that among a group of patients hospitalized due to a heart attack, 69 percent had elevated anxiety scores. Lane and colleagues (2002) found similar results among a group of patients who experienced an acute myocardial infarction. Specifically, they found that over 50 percent of such patients experienced significant levels of anxiety. Further, these heightened symptoms tended to last throughout the first year following the heart attack.

SYMPTOMS OF ACUTE ANXIETY

The following are symptoms of acute anxiety:

- ☐   rapid heart rate

- ☐   feelings of fear or strong apprehension

- ☐   trembling, restlessness, and muscle tension

- ☐   light-headedness or dizziness

- ☐   perspiration, sweating

- ☐   cold hands or feet

- ☐   shortness of breath

- ☐   excessive worry

- ☐   feelings of having little control over events

Anxiety often takes the form of specific fears, especially when you face an immediate threat to your physical or emotional well-being (for example, the fear of harm when driving on snowy roads or the fear of being rejected when asking your boss for a raise). Sometimes, however, anxiety can be aroused in response to dangers that are relatively remote or vague, such as a terrorist attack or getting sick by shaking people's hands. Anxiety that is out of proportion to actual events is one hallmark of an anxiety disorder.

THE DIFFERENT TYPES OF ANXIETY DISORDERS

Examples of excessive or inappropriate anxiety include panic attacks, phobias, and generalized anxiety disorder. *Panic attacks* are brief, intense episodes of anxiety that often occur in the absence of a threatening event. In addition to the symptoms listed above, people experiencing panic attacks may have fears of dying or losing control and may have chills or hot flashes, nausea, or a sensation of choking. Research has found a large overlap between coronary artery disease and *panic disorder,* and panic disorder has further been linked to reduced heart rate variability and myocardial ischemia (Fleet, Lavoie, and Beitman 2000).

Phobias are persistent fears of specific objects or situations. Objects can include such things as snakes, blood, or dogs. Examples of situations include social events, giving a speech in public, or being in tall buildings or enclosed places (such as tunnels or airplanes). *Generalized anxiety disorder* is a more diffuse or nonspecific type of anxiety involving excessive worrying, restlessness, and persistent tension.

Additional types of anxiety disorders involve reactions to traumatic events. These include *acute stress disorder* and *post-traumatic stress disorder*. Both begin when you experience, witness, or are confronted by an event that involves death or serious harm to yourself or others. Both disorders involve reexperiencing the event through thoughts, dreams, or flashbacks; increased arousal and tension; avoidance of certain things related to the event; and a negative impact on your day-to-day functioning. With acute stress disorder, these symptoms appear within one month of the event, whereas with post-traumatic stress disorder, these symptoms can emerge months or years after the event.

A final type of anxiety disorder, *obsessive-compulsive disorder,* involves either significant *obsessions* (that is, recurrent and persistent thoughts, impulses, or images, such as repeated doubts about having left the door unlocked or thoughts of having become contaminated) or *compulsions* (that is, repetitive behaviors, such as persistent handwashing or checking). Such symptoms are problematic when they cause either significant distress or difficulty in day-to-day functioning.

Your Anxiety Symptoms

The anxiety disorders we've just described can be accurately diagnosed only by a professional. But you can assume that you are experiencing significant anxiety if you have three or more of the symptoms listed earlier in this chapter under "Symptoms of Acute Anxiety." To identify your symptoms, go back to that list and check off the ones that are troubling to you. You will use this list later in this chapter to determine which tools will be helpful for your particular symptoms of anxiety.

To track changes in your level of anxiety, first calculate your baseline score on the anxiety section of the "Feelings Test" in chapter 2 by adding up your Yes answers to questions 5, 8, 9, 16, 20, 21, 24, 26, 28, 30, 31, and 33. Then retake this section of the "Feelings Test" after you've been using the self-help tools in this book for about a month. The change in your score will show the progress you've made in managing your anxiety symptoms.

ANXIETY AND HEART DISEASE

Like depression, anxiety not only contributes to the initial development of heart problems, but it also increases your risk of further problems—or even death—if you already have heart disease (Kubzansky et al. 1998).

Anxiety as a Risk Factor for Initial Heart Disease

Several large-scale epidemiologic studies have followed groups of individuals over time in order to determine whether certain characteristics predicted who experienced heart disease and who did not. For example, a ten-year follow-up study of approximately 1,500 men in England demonstrated that symptoms of anxiety reported at baseline were highly predictive of fatal coronary heart disease, even after controlling for other cardiovascular risk factors (Haines, Imeson, and Meade 1987). In fact, phobic anxiety was associated with a 300 percent increase in risk for fatal and nonfatal negative cardiac events, even in people with no preexisting heart disease.

Kawachi, Colditz, and colleagues (1994) conducted another large-scale study, this time following close to 40,000 male health professionals. All individuals were free of heart disease at the beginning of the investigation. These researchers found that the higher a person's level of anxiety, the more likely that person was to experience sudden cardiac death eventually. Similar findings were identified using the Normative Aging Study database established by the Veterans Administration (Kawachi, Sparrow, et al. 1994). Specifically, although no increased risks due to anxiety were found for nonfatal myocardial infarctions or angina, elevated anxiety scores at baseline were associated with an increased risk for sudden cardiac death. In addition, this study identified a significant relationship between worry, a cognitive symptom of anxiety, and the onset of cardiovascular disease.

In a study that focused on female homemakers, Eaker, Pinsky, and Castelli (1992) followed 749 women who were initially healthy for a period of twenty years. Baseline reports of tension and anxiety in this population were found to be strong and independent predictors of coronary heart disease.

Clearly, these studies demonstrate that anxiety is significantly related to the onset of heart disease in initially disease-free individuals and thus is an important risk factor to address.

Anxiety and the Risk of Further Heart Problems

Several studies have been conducted indicating that anxiety can worsen the health outcome of patients who have already experienced some form of cardiovascular disease. For example, Moser and Dracup (1996) found that higher levels of anxiety were associated with increased rates of in-hospital complications, including *reinfarction* (that is, having another heart attack), recurrent ischemia, and ventricular tachycardia and fibrillation. Their results suggested that heart patients with a high level of anxiety during their hospital stay had an almost 500 percent increase in the risk for additional adverse cardiovascular events and death as compared to heart patients without high levels of anxiety. In-hospital anxiety assessed early on was one of the strongest predictors for subsequent in-hospital complications.

Frasure-Smith, Lespérance, and Talajic (1995) found that anxiety significantly predicted recurrent cardiac events over the course of a twelve-month period following a heart attack. In fact, they identified a 250 percent increase in risk for ischemic complications resulting from anxiety following the heart attack.

Anxiety has also been found to trigger ventricular arrhythmias. For example, Lampert and colleagues (2002) asked patients who had an implantable cardioverter defibrillator to record what they were feeling and doing before they received a shock from the device. As you learned in chapter 3, when the ICD detects an abnormally fast heart rate (that is, ventricular tachycardia), it shocks the heart to restore it to a normal rhythm in order to prevent sudden cardiac death. These researchers found that 20 percent of the shocks were preceded by feelings of anxiety, indicating that this negative emotion is a strong risk factor for abnormal heart rhythms.

Furthermore, receiving an ICD shock is often described by people who have this device as similar to being kicked by a horse. For some of these individuals, such a shock can be a very stressful event in itself, potentially leading to the development of post-traumatic stress disorder. This reaction can begin a vicious cycle in which increased anxiety leads you to receive a shock and the experience of receiving a shock increases your overall anxiety. If you have an ICD device, you will want to be especially vigilant about managing your anxiety. You can avoid this cycle—or break out of it—using the strategies we offer in this book.

How Does Anxiety Lead to Heart Disease?

Based on research with both animals and humans, physicians and scientists have developed theories about how anxiety can biologically lead to heart disease.

Anxiety can lead to unhealthy lifestyle habits. It is often associated with loss of sleep, decreased activity, poor diet, and increased tobacco, alcohol, and drug use. As we noted in chapter 3, such behaviors serve as risk factors by themselves for cardiovascular disease.

Some scientists suggest that the link between anxiety and heart disease involves the increases in sympathetic nervous system activity and the release of excess chemical neurotransmitters, such as dopamine and norepinephrine, that occur as a person experiences acute anxiety (Schneiderman 1987). Anxiety can potentially lead to damage to the endothelium (lining) of coronary arteries. Platelets gather at the site of damage; smooth muscle cells proliferate, contributing to the buildup of plaque; and excess fatty acids are released and deposited at the site of damage. Together, these three processes can restrict blood flow to the heart (Carney et al. 2002; Musselman et al. 1996).

Anxiety can also cause narrowing of the arteries because it increases blood pressure and heart rate. Studies have shown that anxiety can increase a man's risk for hypertension by 250 percent (Markovitz et al. 1993). In another investigation, Markovitz and colleagues (1991) found that women who initially had normal blood pressure levels were more likely to have increases in their systolic blood pressure if they also reported anxiety at baseline.

Anxiety can also promote hardening of the arteries through *hyperlipidemia,* or the elevation of lipids in the blood. In a review of the relevant scientific literature, Hayward (1995) found a consistent link between anxiety and high cholesterol levels.

Scientists also suggest that anxiety can lead to heart disease as a function of its negative effects on the electrical stability of the heart. Anxiety can influence electrical instability, potentially leading to ventricular arrhythmias (Lown 1987). Anxiety may also predispose a person to *ventricular premature beats,* which have been identified as a risk factor for electrical instability and sudden cardiac death (Kubzansky et al. 1998).

Anxiety has also been found to be linked to low heart rate variability (Kawachi et al. 1995). Generally, greater variability in heart rate is associated with good cardiovascular health, because the variability buffers the negative cardiovascular effects of stress. Reduced HRV is a risk factor for sudden cardiac death and tends to be associated with poor cardiovascular health (Gorman and Sloan 2000).

The *vagus nerve* is one of twelve pairs of cranial nerves that lead directly from the brain to other parts of the body. Besides controlling swallowing, speech, and the gag reflex, the vagus nerve also controls the muscles of the heart. In general, low vagal control of the heart rate has been linked with both life-threatening arrhythmias and sudden cardiac death. Watkins and colleagues (1998) found anxiety to be strongly associated with reductions in vagal control of the heart.

Collectively, it would seem that anxiety can lead to a variety of heart problems through a variety of pathways or mechanisms of action.

ANXIETY CAN BE EFFECTIVELY TREATED

Like depression, anxiety can be effectively treated. Both antianxiety (or *anxiolytic*) medication and certain forms of psychotherapy and counseling have been found to be highly effective. Research has shown that cognitive behavioral therapy techniques, such as cognitive therapy, stress management strategies, behavioral activation, problem-solving therapy, and self-control therapy, are especially effective in treating anxiety (Nezu, Nezu, and Lombardo 2004). The strategies we'll teach you in this book are based on cognitive behavioral therapy.

Significantly, research has found that counseling programs based on such strategies are effective not only for reducing anxiety but also for reducing various underlying biologically related risk factors. For example, Blumenthal and colleagues (1997) found that a cognitive behavioral stress management program reduced myocardial ischemia among patients with coronary heart disease. In addition, a review of the literature regarding the effectiveness of Transcendental Meditation programs found that this type of meditation consistently led to decreases in blood pressure, artery blockages, myocardial ischemia, *left ventricular hypertrophy* (enlargement of the left ventricle), and mortality (Walton et al. 2002). Dean Ornish (1996) developed a program that has been found to be highly effective for reversing heart disease. In addition to prescribing a certain heart-healthy diet, Ornish's program emphasizes many of the same counseling and self-help strategies, such as breathing and relaxation exercises, that we'll teach you in this guidebook.

WHAT YOU CAN DO NOW ABOUT YOUR ANXIETY

The self-help strategies contained in this book will help you better manage your anxiety symptoms. You can begin by learning the types of tools you identified in the "What Is

Your Tool Chest Profile?" exercise in chapter 2 as being especially suited to you. Alternatively, you can use the table below to match your symptoms with the tools that are typically most effective in managing those symptoms.

Symptom	Related Tools
worry or fear about realistic problems	"Enhancing Positive Experiences" (chapter 11) "Solving Stressful Problems" (chapter 13) "Getting Social Support" (chapter 19) "Awakening Your Spirituality" (chapter 20)
unrealistic fears (worries about events that are unlikely to happen)	"Using Feelings to Better Know Yourself" (chapter 7) "Expressing Emotions Constructively" (chapter 8) "Changing Negative Thinking" (chapter 12) "Visualizing Success" (chapter 18) "Getting Social Support" (chapter 19) "Awakening Your Spirituality" (chapter 20)
physical symptoms	"Using Feelings to Better Know Yourself" (chapter 7) "Expressing Emotions Constructively" (chapter 8) "Deep Breathing" (chapter 14) "Autogenic Training" (chapter 15) "Deep Muscle Relaxation" (chapter 16) "Mind Travel to a Safe Place" (chapter 17)

YOUR PERSONAL PLAN FOR ANXIETY

In your notebook or journal, write down your personal plan to help reduce your anxiety. Begin by choosing at least three tools. Make a commitment to learn them to the best of your ability. Remember that as with all other skills, like driving a car or playing a sport, practice over time is required to get better. Don't get discouraged!

You may want to add to your list of tools. The more tools you use, the more likely you are to be successful in managing your anxiety. Remember to track your progress, be persistent, actively read each relevant chapter, and reward yourself for success.

6

Anger and Heart Disease

We all get angry and annoyed at times. The plumber doesn't come when he promised. The car in front of you is going too slow. The pottery you ordered and waited six weeks for finally comes in the mail but is broken when you open it. Your pet soils your new rug minutes before company arrives. You find out that your son or daughter lied to you about smoking cigarettes. You don't get the raise you feel you deserve. The people sitting behind you at the movies will not stop talking. The cashier at the grocery store is talking nonstop with a friend and ignores you as you wait. While you're standing on the curb during a big downpour, a taxi drives by and splashes you all over with puddle water. Need we go on?

Of course, many of these situations would make any person mad. But for how long, how intensely, and how frequently? The answers determine whether your angry reactions are essentially harmless or whether you are experiencing what psychologist Doyle Gentry (2000) calls "toxic anger." He defines toxic anger as more frequent, more intense, and longer lasting than simple annoyance and frustration. People experiencing such levels of anger often express it overtly (for example, by throwing a book at the family pet) and tend to be defensive. Toxic anger is usually unreasonable given the situation and is generally uncontrollable (that is, difficult to stop once it gets started).

IS TOXIC ANGER BAD FOR YOU?

Is this type of anger harmful? Consider the title of the book written by internist and psychiatrist Redford Williams and his wife, Virginia: *Anger Kills* (1993). This title is not an exaggeration. Williams spent decades researching the role of anger in cardiovascular health and concluded that anger and hostility have significant negative effects on heart health. Research relating anger to heart disease began over thirty years ago when two cardiologists, Meyer Friedman and Ray Rosenman, documented a strong association between what they called "type A personality" and coronary heart disease (Rosenman et al. 1975). Specifically, individuals who were initially healthy and were classified as type A were found to be more than twice as likely to have coronary heart disease eight and a half years later as people without the type A behavioral patterns.

Type A personality traits were originally defined as always being in a hurry, easily becoming hostile and angry, having a high need for control, and being very competitive and ambitious. Although further scientific studies documented the significant relationship between type A behavior and CHD, a finer analysis indicated that the characteristics of being hurried, impatient, and achievement oriented were not the critical components, but that anger and hostility were the factors responsible for the association with heart disease (Rozanski, Blumenthal, and Kaplan 1999).

ANGER, AGGRESSION, AND HOSTILITY

What is the difference between anger and aggression? Between anger and hostility? *Anger* is an emotional state that is associated with specific thoughts and physical symptoms. *Aggression* is overt behavior showing an intent to do harm or injury to a person or object. *Hostility* is a trait of anger that occurs across many different types of situations and is often combined with verbal or physical aggression.

Looking closely at these definitions, there appear to be three major components to this negative emotion:

- physiological arousal and feelings of anger (getting hot under the collar, feeling like your head is about to explode, feeling your temperature rise)

- angry or hostile thoughts (*I wish this person would just shut up and go away. I'll show him who's the boss! You can't trust anybody!*)

- aggressive acts (cutting someone off on the road, shoving someone who makes fun of you, kicking a dog)

However, you don't have to have all three to be experiencing toxic levels of anger.

What are your symptoms of anger and hostility? Look over your answers to the "Feelings Test" in chapter 2. Do you find yourself getting angry frequently and have physical symptoms of anger (for example, Yes answers to questions 6 and 15)? If so, check off the category "feelings of anger or negative arousal" below. If you often have anger-related thoughts (for example, Yes answers to questions 11 and 19), check that category. If you experience urges to harm someone or something, or have found yourself actually engaging in such actions (for example, Yes answers to questions 22 and 25), then check off the "aggressive wishes or behavior" category. Checking off these symptoms will be helpful later in this chapter when we outline which tools are helpful for which symptoms of anger and hostility.

☐   feelings of anger or negative arousal

☐   angry or hostile thinking

☐   aggressive wishes or behavior

Add up your Yes answers on the anger section of the "Feelings Test" in chapter 2 (questions 3, 4, 6, 11, 12, 15, 18, 19, 22, 25, 27, and 29). This is your baseline score. After about a month of using the self-help tools you choose from this book, retake this section of the test. Your new score will show the progress you've made in managing your anger and hostility.

ANGER, HOSTILITY, AND HEART DISEASE

Persistent anger and hostility have been found to increase vulnerability to heart disease (Sirois and Burg 2003). Like depression and anxiety, anger and hostility can contribute to the development of initial heart problems and can increase your risk for further problems if you are already experiencing some type of heart disease.

Anger as a Risk Factor for Initial Heart Disease

Numerous investigations have demonstrated the relationship between anger and the development of CHD. For example, Kawachi and colleagues (1996) followed over 1,300 men who participated in the Normative Aging Study. Upon entering the study, individuals were asked about symptoms ranging from mild irritation to episodes of intense anger that involved aggression and violent acts. Over the course of the next seven years, those individuals who reported the highest levels of anger at baseline were found to be over 250 percent more likely to experience CHD events than men reporting the lowest levels of anger.

Everson and colleagues (1997) studied over 2,000 men to determine the increased risk of cardiovascular mortality related to hostility. These investigators found that men who had hostility scores in the top quarter among this sample were at more than twice the risk of cardiovascular mortality—and death from any cause—compared to men with hostility scores in the lowest quarter. Among those individuals without any previous myocardial infarction or angina, high hostility scorers also had a 200 percent increased risk of an initial heart attack.

In a study that included close to 3,000 men in South Wales, symptoms of anger, as well as anger suppression, significantly predicted the incidence of ischemic heart disease, even after controlling for physiological risk factors such as blood pressure, cholesterol levels, smoking, alcohol consumption, and caloric intake (Gallacher et al. 1999).

Chang and colleagues (2002) found that among a sample of over 1,000 men between the ages of thirty-two and forty-eight, those who responded angrily to stressful events were three and a half to six and a half times more likely to suffer premature cardiovascular disease, CHD, and heart attacks than individuals with low levels of anger.

Analyzing data from close to 13,000 people as part of the Atherosclerosis Risk in Communities Study, Williams and colleagues (2000) found that a person who is prone to anger is about three times more likely to have a heart attack or sudden cardiac death compared to an individual who is not anger prone. These findings were true even after taking into account the presence of other risk factors, such as cigarette smoking, diabetes, cholesterol, and obesity.

Eaker and colleagues (2004) reported that among a sample of 3,873 adults who participated in the Framingham Offspring Study from 1984 to 1987, symptoms of anger and hostility were significant and independent predictors of *atrial fibrillation* (that is, abnormal contractions of the upper chambers of the heart) in men. Moreover, anger was also predictive of total mortality in men.

Research has also demonstrated that physiologically, hostile individuals respond differently than nonhostile people to stressful and anger-provoking situations. For example, Smith and Gallo (1999) found that hostile men, in reaction to a stressful interaction with their spouse, responded with greater systolic blood pressure. Hostile individuals, in reliving a self-chosen anger memory, had larger and longer-lasting blood pressure responses as compared to nonhostile people (Fredrickson et al. 2000). Möller and colleagues (1999) found strong evidence that an episode of intense anger can actually trigger a heart attack, and the increased risk lasts for approximately one hour after the outburst of anger. Mittleman and colleagues (1995) found similar results among a sample of over 1,600 heart patients.

These studies clearly demonstrate that anger and hostility are significantly associated with the onset of heart disease in initially disease-free individuals, suggesting that they are important risk factors to address.

Anger and the Risk of Further Heart Problems

Research has also documented that anger and hostility can worsen the health outcome of patients already experiencing some type of heart problem. For example, among a group of 3,750 Finnish men aged forty to fifty-nine, high levels of irritability and quickness to anger were significantly related to increased CHD mortality for those individuals with preexisting heart disease (Koskenvuo et al. 1988). Hecker and colleagues (1988) compared a group of patients with CHD with control subjects and found that hostility was associated with a close to 200 percent increase in risk for cardiac death, subsequent heart attacks, and chest pain. Patients with CHD and high hostility scores were found to be two and a half times more likely to experience *restenosis* (that is, narrowing of the arteries again after balloon angioplasty), as compared to CHD patients low in hostility (Goodman et al. 1996).

In addition, CHD patients with high hostility scores have been found to be at a 200 percent increased risk for other cardiac problems (Mendes de Leon et al. 1996), show more rapid atherosclerosis (Julkumen et al. 1994), and show more ischemia during stress testing (Helmers et al. 1993). Matthews and colleagues (2004) reported that high levels of hostility were associated with a greater mortality rate among a group of men who were initially identified as being at high risk for CHD due to other factors (for example, high cholesterol levels, high blood pressure, and cigarette smoking) as compared to their nonhostile (but high risk for CHD) counterparts. Lampert and colleagues (2002) demonstrated that anger can actually trigger ventricular arrhythmias in patients with an implantable cardioverter defibrillator. Gabbay and colleagues (1996) found that anger led to increased ischemia (that is, reduced blood flow) and greater heart rates among a sample of CHD patients. Last, among a group of patients with coronary artery disease, we found that when they recalled an angry incident, they had significant increases in systolic blood pressure and problems with the functioning of the heart's left ventricle (Jain et al. 2001).

How Do Anger and Hostility Lead to Heart Disease?

Like depression and anxiety, anger and hostility can lead to increased cigarette smoking, poor diet, obesity, and alcoholism. Such behavioral risk factors by themselves are vulnerability factors for cardiovascular disease.

Anger and hostility can lead to heart disease through chronic overstimulation of the sympathetic nervous system (Keefe, Castell, and Blumenthal 1986). For example, in general, hostile individuals manifest higher heart rate and blood pressure responses to environmental stressors, including mental tasks (Sul and Wan 1993). They also respond to day-to-day activities with higher blood pressure levels (Suarez and Blumenthal 1991). This overstimulation can lead to the release of excess *plasma catecholamines* (that is, chemical neurotransmitters, such as dopamine and norepinephrine), which can lead to damage of the endothelium of coronary arteries. This can lead to the release of excess fatty acids, platelet aggregation, smooth muscle proliferation, and the deposit of lipids at the site of the endothelium damage. It can also lead to arterial constriction, increased blood pressure and heart rate, and increased ventricular dysfunctions (Rozanski, Blumenthal, and Kaplan 1999).

Low control of the heart rate by the vagus nerve has been associated with both life-threatening arrhythmias and sudden cardiac death. Sloan and colleagues (1994) found that the higher a person's level of hostility, the lower that person's vagal control of the heart. In addition, Brosschot and Thayer (1998) suggest that attempts to suppress anger can also lead to ineffective vagal functioning.

Anger and hostility can reduce blood flow to the brain. Shapiro and colleagues (2000), for example, compared adult men high in hostility to low-hostility men and found that in reaction to a mentally stressful task (rapid serial subtraction by sevens beginning with a four-digit number), highly hostile individuals had greater increases in heart rate and greater decreases in heart rate variability. Moreover, in highly hostile men, this stressful task led to reduced blood flow to the *prefrontal cortex* (that part of the brain associated with social behavior). Damage to the prefrontal cortex is usually characterized by aggressive outbursts, argumentative behavior, loss of self-control, and poor social judgment. Thus the link between hostility and cardiovascular disease may involve the negative effects on certain parts of the brain.

TOXIC ANGER CAN BE EFFECTIVELY TREATED

Toxic anger is treatable. A recent review of the scientific literature regarding anger management or anger reduction counseling programs strongly underscores their effectiveness (Del Vecchio and O'Leary 2004). Cognitive behavioral therapy has been shown to be effective with large numbers of patients with various anger problems (Nezu, Nezu, and Lombardo 2004). The tools in this book are based on this scientifically supported form of psychotherapy.

Several studies have specifically demonstrated the effectiveness of anger reduction techniques for cardiac patients. Larkin and Zayfert (1996) found that a cognitive behavioral anger management program led to significant reductions in diastolic blood pressure for a group of patients diagnosed with essential hypertension. In addition, relaxation training (like the tools we'll teach in chapters 14, 15, and 16) was found to reduce blood pressure reactivity to an anger-instigating situation for patients with borderline hypertension. In a similar study, Davison and colleagues (1992) found that relaxation therapy led to significant reductions in blood pressure and heart rate and that reductions in anger and hostility were strongly correlated with these cardiovascular improvements.

Burell and colleagues (1994) examined the effects of a psychosocial counseling program on type A behavior among a group of men who previously had a heart attack. Patients receiving such treatment were found to experience significant reductions in type A behavior and anger; they also had improved medical outcomes and fewer recurrences of negative cardiac events.

The Recurrent Coronary Prevention Project was designed to reduce type A behavioral patterns among a sample of over 1,000 post–heart attack patients (Thoresen and Bracke 1997). Patients receiving cognitive behavioral counseling not only experienced marked reductions in type A behaviors but also experienced a significantly lower rate of coronary recurrence compared to heart patients receiving ordinary psychoeducation. Close to eight and a half years after treatment, patients who received the type A intervention continued to demonstrate significantly reduced levels of hostility and anger, highlighting the long-term success of such a program.

In a well-controlled investigation, Gidron, Davidson, and Bata (1999) evaluated the efficacy of a cognitive behavioral intervention for a group of men with CHD and high hostility. In general, compared to similarly hostile CHD patients not receiving this program, treated patients were found to experience significant reductions in blood pressure after two months. Moreover, these improvements to cardiovascular health were found to be significantly related to reductions in hostility.

Collectively, these scientific studies suggest that psychosocial counseling programs can reduce anger and hostility. But more importantly to you, they also appear to have the ability to improve heart health.

WHAT YOU CAN DO NOW ABOUT YOUR ANGER

The self-help strategies we'll teach you in this book will help you reduce your levels of hostility and anger. You can begin by learning the types of tools you decided would suit you best in the "What Is Your Tool Chest Profile?" exercise in chapter 2. You can also use the table below to match the aspect of anger that you identified earlier in this chapter as being most troublesome to you with the tools that are most effective in addressing that aspect.

Components of Anger	Related Tools
feelings of anger or negative arousal	"Using Feelings to Better Know Yourself" (chapter 7) "Expressing Emotions Constructively" (chapter 8) "Deep Breathing" (chapter 14) "Autogenic Training" (chapter 15) "Deep Muscle Relaxation" (chapter 16) "Mind Travel to a Safe Place" (chapter 17) "Awakening Your Spirituality" (chapter 20)
angry or hostile thinking	"Expressing Emotions Constructively" (chapter 8) "Fostering Acceptance" (chapter 9) "Learning to Forgive" (chapter 10) "Changing Negative Thinking" (chapter 12) "Awakening Your Spirituality" (chapter 20)
aggressive wishes or behaviors	"Getting Social Support" (chapter 19) "Awakening Your Spirituality" (chapter 20)

YOUR PERSONAL PLAN FOR ANGER

Take out your notebook or journal and write down your personal plan to help reduce your anger or feelings of hostility. Include at least three tools to try first. Make a commitment to yourself to learn the techniques and practice them diligently. Once you've learned the first few tools, try some new ones. Remember that the more tools you use, the more likely you are to succeed. Don't forget to be an active reader, be persistent and practice often, track your progress, and reward yourself as you reach your goals.

Part 3

Coping with
Negative Emotions

7

Emotional Tool: Using Feelings to Better Know Yourself

"How ya doing?" is a very common greeting among people when they meet. A very typical answer is "Fine, thanks. How 'bout you?" It is conventional wisdom that when talking with acquaintances or coworkers, or when meeting people for the first time, a neutral response is actually appropriate. However, such a response is so commonplace that people tend to answer that way automatically, even when they are experiencing some discomfort. If you respond this way chronically, without paying attention to what you are really feeling, you can actually lose touch with your emotions.

Moreover, when people experience a negative emotion such as fear, anger, sadness, guilt, or embarrassment, they often want to get rid of the feeling as quickly as possible. We remember one heart patient, Pete, who told us that he felt negative emotions were silly because they don't solve problems. When we asked if he actually feels negative emotions like sadness, tension, or anger, he replied that he does, but added, "What's the use in harping on them?" Pete explained that his father always told him, "Just deal with life and be a man! Just do what you have to, and don't whine about it." Unfortunately, Pete came to believe this meant that any time he felt any negative emotion, no matter what type or how intense, he needed to suppress the feelings because they were "useless."

Ironically, research has shown that emotional suppression not only fails to provide relief from that emotion but actually interferes with successful adaptation and coping. Further, it can lead to widespread increases in activation of the sympathetic nervous system related to cardiovascular functioning (Gross and Levenson 1997). Simply put, suppressing emotions can have harmful effects on your heart. For example, attempts to suppress even the minor emotion of embarrassment lead to increases in both systolic and diastolic blood pressures (Harris 2001). In addition, this same research suggests that the longer you attempt to suppress an emotion, the more physiologically demanding it becomes to do so, taking a greater toll on your body.

FEELINGS ARE THE WINDOW TO YOUR HEART

Do you tend to try to downplay your emotions? If so, you may be missing many opportunities to know yourself better. Desire to suppress an emotion can make you forget that feelings can actually increase your insight and can provide you with a very important view into your heart and soul. Psychologists consider feelings to be precious tools because they serve as cues to stop and become aware of the underlying emotions. Through this process of awareness, upsetting feelings can actually help people better understand what changes are important to consider, more effectively set personal goals, and improve their quality of life.

In this chapter, we'll present a step-by-step approach that will help you to

- increase your understanding that feelings—even powerful or upsetting ones—are normal,

- better recognize your own feelings when they occur,

- use your emotions to work for you and your well-being,

- know what is important to you, and

- set personal goals.

People experience distressing feelings every day. Sometimes feelings are a reaction to a single situation or thought, and they simply pass. For example, you may become angry and frustrated when you are stuck in a morning traffic jam. However, the feeling is fleeting and does not occur all the time. On the other hand, you may be bothered by upsetting feelings for a long period of time. For example, you may experience repeated feelings of hurt or anger in certain relationships or have chronic fears about injury or illness. Problems like depression, anxiety, anger, and bereavement all involve distressful feelings that are sometimes difficult to change.

The feelings may be even more troublesome if you experience several different emotions at the same time or fail to recognize your feelings. For example, you may believe that you are angry when in fact you are feeling sad or scared. Moreover, you may regret the way you express or communicate your feelings to other people. For example, some people become very quiet and unresponsive to their spouse or partner when they are feeling sad or preoccupied with fears. In such cases, others often misinterpret this withdrawn behavior as rejecting, hurtful, or uncaring. Suppressing feelings can even have a negative effect on your ability to process information (Gross and Levenson 1997).

In addition, some people try to block out or avoid upsetting emotions by withdrawing socially or abusing drugs or alcohol. Unfortunately, these are only quick-fix solutions that temporarily take you away from your feelings.

If you have experienced difficulties like these in how you cope with distressing feelings, then this chapter is likely to be very helpful to you. There are much more effective ways to use the negative feelings that you experience. That's the purpose of this tool. If you experience confusing or distressful emotions (and we know you do simply because you are human), then this tool is especially important for you.

This exercise is designed to give a step-by-step approach so you can use the power of feelings to your advantage. By practicing these steps, you will become more aware of your negative feelings and learn to use them as the window to your heart, creating a deeper understanding about the person you want to be. Instead of avoiding or running away from your feelings, you will come to value them as a precious instrument with which you can see into your heart. We all experience negative feelings. Rather than simply allowing them to continue to make you feel bad, use them to your advantage!

USING FEELINGS TO BETTER KNOW YOURSELF

First, take out your journal. Record the information requested in each step. Begin each entry by noting the date and time. The following are the pieces of information that you should jot down in your journal. We'll explain them in more detail below.

1. Notice feelings when they happen.

2. Stop and become aware of the feeling.

3. Record your level of emotional distress.

4. Describe the feelings you experienced.

5. Listen to the information you learned by paying attention to your feelings.

Step 1: Notice feelings when they happen

Throughout the day, anytime you begin to feel upset or distressed, stop and notice what you are feeling and how intense it is. Imagine that this emotion is providing a special view of what is really important to you. Then put the feeling into words. Rather than trying to get rid of it, remember that this is an important opportunity to get to know yourself better. Get out your journal and write down the emotions you are experiencing as soon as you are able.

Step 2: Stop and be aware of the feeling

Here is your chance to open the window to your heart. Imagine a stop sign or a flashing red traffic light signaling you to stop. This means stopping *all* action, as if you have pressed the pause button on a video player or movie camera. You are going to stop all actions (even talking) for a few seconds to listen to the feeling you have identified and written down. In this frozen moment in time, you should complete steps three through five.

Step 3: Record your distress level

In this step, you simply record your emotional distress level. This will help you experience the intensity and focus on how you're feeling in the moment, and it will also give you a way to monitor your progress. Use a scale from 1 to 10, where 1 represents total peace of mind and tranquillity and 10 is the most distressed you could possibly become. Give your current distress a number from 1 to 10 right now.

Step 4: Describe the feelings

Now think about the important information that you are receiving from your emotions. This step is geared to help you open the window into your heart—in other words, to better understand what your emotions are allowing you to see and hear. This can be hard work, because it means giving yourself the time to figure out what important information your feelings are providing you. With this new insight, however, even distressful emotions can be a gift—a powerful tool that will help you understand yourself better. More importantly, having this insight allows you to think about why you are having this feeling and how you want to address the problems that you are facing.

Think about where you experience this feeling the most. Do you have physical sensations, like your heart pounding, a lump in your throat, or your face flushing? Do you say things to yourself like *I can't take this, I feel so alone, No one understands me, They don't care,* or *I give up*? As you begin to get familiar with how you experience your own emotions, consider all of these signs (that is, both the physical sensations and the things you say to yourself) as clues to what your heart has to say to you.

Step 5: Listen to the feelings

Now you are ready to listen to your feelings and write down the information that your feelings are providing. Practicing this part is an important way that you can develop insight. Remember why you have emotions in the first place: to give you information. Your body is hardwired to react with certain feelings for very good reasons. Consider the following examples:

■ You experience fear when there is a danger to which you must react in order to keep safe.

■ You experience anger when you want something but feel thwarted in your efforts to get what you want. You must figure out another way to get closer to what you want, or you must ask yourself if what you want is as important as you perceive it to be.

■ You experience sadness when you lose something or someone and must accept a change of some kind.

■ You experience a combination of anxiety, anger, and sadness when another person or situation is responsible for your fear or loss.

Your goal is to try to change the "software" to allow yourself to gain insight into what your emotions are trying to tell you.

LISTENING TO FEELINGS: WHAT YOUR EMOTIONS SAY TO YOU

The last step can be difficult, so we'll give you some further guidance about the type of information you should be looking for when you are trying to listen to your feelings. We have also provided a few common examples of what the information may reveal. These are examples of the kind of insight you will gain as you learn to pay better attention to your emotions.

Feeling: Fear

Common ways people describe fear: Nervous, jittery, on edge, scared, anxious, restless, uncomfortable, worried, panicked.

Information to look for: Any sense of impending hurt, pain, threat, or danger.

What the information may reveal:

■ You fear physical or emotional injury for yourself or others.

- You fear that you are inferior to others and your sense of self-esteem is threatened (you have fears about your intelligence, talents, physical skill, or outward appearance).

Why this information is important:

- You can now work on better managing your fears rather than trying to avoid them.

- You can examine the fears you have and see if they are realistic. Some of the thinking tools may be very helpful in coping with these fears.

- You can face your fears and work on ways to reduce them. Similar to facing a schoolyard bully, facing your fears often leads to greater self-confidence, even if you sustain a bruise or two.

Feeling: Anger

Common ways people describe anger: Frustrated, irritated, enraged, mad, pissed off, angry, wanting to break something or hurt someone.

Information to look for: Being blocked from getting what you want. The block can be due to circumstances or specific people.

What the information may reveal:

- You want success, achievement, or to be the best, but you see someone or something in the way.

- You want a relationship, but it seems like hard work, or you see the other person as creating problems.

- You want to be loved or admired, but others do not appreciate you.

- You want to be able to control circumstances or the reactions of others, but it is impossible to have that much control over situations or people.

Why the information is important:

- You may discover that your anger is less about the other person and more about yourself, your pride, or what you want. Rather than focusing on your anger, you can direct your energies toward making your own life better.

- You may have unrealistic expectations of others or yourself. It may be time for you to "get real"—to give yourself and others a break from such harsh standards.

Feeling: Sadness

Common ways people describe sadness: Let down, disappointed, devastated, hurt, unhappy, depressed, drained, miserable, downcast, heartbroken.

Information to look for: Losing something or holding the belief that you have lost something or someone important to you.

What the information may reveal:

- You have lost a person (such as a friend, lover, family member, or partner) through a move, illness, death, disagreement, or estrangement, or because the person chooses to be with other people.

- You have lost something other than a person. This may be something tangible (for example, money, job, physical health, leisure time) or something intangible (for example, a role in the family, a position at work, respect from others).

Why the information is important:

- You can begin to work on increasing pleasant or joyful moments in your life to help you heal from a loss. The behavioral action tools may be helpful with this.

- You may have the opportunity to see that your worth is more than the objects you've lost. For example, your wealth is not a measure of your self-esteem; your physical strength is not equal to your spirit.

Feeling: Embarrassment

Common ways people describe embarrassment: humiliated, vulnerable, self-conscious, feel like crawling in a hole.

Information to look for: Revealing your vulnerabilities.

What the information may reveal:

- You are concerned that others can see your imperfections, mistakes, and problems.

Why the information is important:

- You can begin to focus less on imperfection and more on accepting yourself for the person you are.

Feeling: Guilt

Common ways people describe guilt: ashamed, feel bad, screwed up, failed.

Information to look for: You regret something you did.

What the information may reveal:

■   You have hurt others through your own actions.

■   You have not done anything wrong, but you are telling yourself that you were wrong (or someone else is telling you that you were wrong) and you doubt yourself.

Why the information is important:

■   You can work on ways to communicate your regret and make a plan for personal change for the better.

■   In the case of self-doubt, you can begin to change your inner voice such that you do not require the approval of others 100 percent of the time.

WHAT TO DO WITH THE INFORMATION YOU'VE GAINED

The information you gain from paying attention to your emotions can direct you toward the next steps to take. For example, if you are feeling angry, it may be important for you to work on alternative ways to get what you want. Other information may suggest that you must face a new situation or change. For example, you may be frightened because you are moving to a new apartment or house.

Finally, the information your feelings provide may indicate that your mind is engaging in a type of self-talk that is inaccurate but your emotional reactions are based on such thoughts as if they were actually true. For example, you may be sad because of an argument you had with a friend or family member. You feel sad because you are telling yourself that this person no longer cares about you. In such a case, the most effective action may be to work on the accuracy of your own thinking. If your emotions point to a situation where negative *thinking* may be responsible for the negative *feeling* (for example, *I had a disagreement with my friend and now she hates me*), you can use the tools in this book that are designed to help you change negative thinking patterns (see chapter 12). However, if what you are saying to yourself is based upon true facts (for example, you are facing a loss or difficult change), consider using the tools that provide you with ways to increase your joy, enlist social support, or strengthen your spirituality as additional ways to help you get through a difficult time (see chapters 11, 19, and 20).

WORKING WITH YOUR FEELINGS

Once you learn to use your emotions to look into your heart, you can apply more logical thinking to decide what those feelings are saying to you. Trying to avoid them or block them out only makes the situation worse. Your emotions can help you make important decisions about situations that are important to you. Here are a few questions to ask yourself as you listen to your feelings.

Do you need to allow these emotions to occur and pass? If so, allow your negative feelings to stay for a while, and notice them. Do not try to rush them away. Just let them happen and pass. You can do this by sitting quietly and not judging or reacting to your feelings. For example, as you notice a distressful emotion such as sorrow, do not allow your mind to draw any conclusions about the feeling or try to justify it. Simply state to yourself, *I notice that I am feeling sad.* Staying aware of the feeling without further need to react to it allows the time to tolerate the feelings as you listen to them.

Do you need to calm your emotions? Sometimes the feelings are so strong or overwhelming that you may need to calm your body down a bit before you can hear what the feeling has to say. When this is the case, consider using one of the relaxation tools in chapters 14 through 16. They are designed to trigger a calm and tranquil physical state.

Do you need to make a change in your life? If so, the "Enhancing Positive Experiences" tool may be helpful to you.

Are you afraid? It is important to remember that not only are your feelings normal, they are actually precious pieces of information about what is happening to you. In this way, negative emotions are not something to be feared or avoided but something to be tuned in to.

Now that you are beginning to gain a better understanding of what your negative emotions are telling you about yourself and your life, remember that the many other tools in this book can help you to make better decisions about what to do next and how to go about achieving such goals.

8

Emotional Tool: Expressing Emotions Constructively

Emotions are an integral part of being human. Our language is full of colorful phrases that demonstrate our recognition of the breadth and depth of emotional experience, as well as how intimately emotions are tied to physical phenomena. Phrases such as "hot under the collar," "a lump in the throat," "sick from guilt," "letting off steam," "coldhearted," "stunned with grief," "a cold sweat," and "heartbroken" are all part of our day-to-day vocabulary for describing common emotions. The reason these phrases contain descriptions of physical phenomena is that emotions actually involve physical changes, such as a flushed face, changes in heart rate and breathing, cold or warm hands, muscle tension, and changes in gastrointestinal functioning.

In addition to the changes we can actually perceive, there are many physical changes of which we are largely unaware, such as changes in brain activity and the release of certain brain chemicals, an imbalance in hormone levels, or variations in the electrical activity of the heart (Rosenberg et al. 2001; Stowell et al. 2003). In fact, even when you deny or attempt to suppress an emotion, many of these physical changes still occur. When the emotions are intense, traumatic, or frequently triggered, this can result in significant physical changes that exert a toll on any part of the body that is affected by feelings: mental processes, the cardiovascular system, the gastrointestinal system, muscles, and immune functioning. Your biological hardwiring—a function of genetic inheritance—determines those parts of the body that are most likely to be affected.

WHY IT IS IMPORTANT TO EXPRESS EMOTIONS

We know from the work of many behavioral scientists that expressing distressing emotions such as anger, sadness, or fear in written and verbal form can have a profound impact on a person's well-being. In fact, psychologists have developed expressive therapies to help people reduce the harmful effects of negative emotions on their physical and mental health. Expressive psychological therapies include techniques that are designed to increase a person's awareness and constructive expression of feelings. *Written emotional disclosure*, for example, refers to writing about thoughts and feelings with regard to a personally stressful and traumatic event. This type of expressive therapy has consistently demonstrated positive effects on mood, physical functioning, and general well-being. Scientific studies conducted by researchers who specialize in how the mind and body interact regarding health and illness have shown that when you experience strong and distressing emotional reactions, putting them into words can serve to organize your thinking, make some sense of what you want to change in yourself or in your life situations, and enhance your ability to remain open and optimistic. The very act of communicating your deepest and most private feelings in a safe and nonjudgmental environment to a listener whom you perceive as wise, understanding, and caring can have very healing and therapeutic effects for both emotional and physical pain.

Research conducted by psychologist James Pennebaker (1995) and others has shown that emotional disclosure results in greater positive mood, less negative mood (such as anxiety), fewer negative physical symptoms, and fewer physician visits. Although many therapists believe that having patients disclose their feelings makes them better able to manage their thoughts and feelings concerning distressing events, they differ in their explanation of *why* writing or talking about such events or persistent feelings seems to be important to a person's mental and physical health. Some believe, based on conditioning theory, that the more you "expose" yourself to a stressful topic or situation, the more you become accustomed to your thoughts and feelings about it. This process is known as *habituation*. Your body becomes so used to reacting to the event that it no longer reacts with distress. Others propose that when people repress or inhibit emotional reactions or stressful memories (for example, purposefully not thinking about their negative thoughts and feelings), they exert significant mental and physical energy, and the feelings continue to resurface. This energy drain can have psychological, emotional, and medical consequences. Regardless of why emotional disclosure works, the important point to remember is that it *does* work.

There are many studies that measure physical stress responses when people either share or hold back their thoughts and feelings about a stressful event. These studies support the idea that confronting stressful events through writing or speaking about them can enhance your understanding and acceptance of distressing events and feelings and decrease your need to hold back and inhibit your thoughts about them. As a result, you experience improvement in both physical and emotional health (Wenzlaff and Wegner 2002).

The "Expressing Emotions Constructively" tool will give you the opportunity to use the technique of emotional disclosure when you are confronting stressful emotions or having difficulty coping with life situations. For this exercise, you will need to have materials available in order to write down your thoughts. You can write on pieces of paper, use a private diary or journal, or type your thoughts on your personal computer. All of these alternatives will work equally well. You should be prepared to write for about twenty minutes. We suggest that you practice this technique once a week for three weeks, then take a break from the practice and assess both your mood and the usefulness of the tool.

EXPRESSING EMOTIONS CONSTRUCTIVELY

The following steps will help you learn to express your emotions in a way that is constructive and heart-healthy.

Step 1: Find a private place to write down your feelings

Take out your writing materials and find a quiet place where you will be free of distractions (for example, children, other people, telephone calls). You will need approximately twenty minutes to complete this task, and you should not be interrupted. When you are seated and ready to begin, set a timer or alarm clock for twenty minutes or note the time on your watch.

Step 2: Write down your feelings

Describe how you are feeling and the situation that led to your feeling this way. You may write about a current incident or a past event. Sometimes current incidents trigger thoughts of very emotionally upsetting incidents or situations that occurred in the past. Whether the situation is new or old, it is important that you choose one that is upsetting or traumatic. Only you know what is truly upsetting to you. Common topics include the death of a loved one, the breakup of a romantic relationship, a major disappointment, or a personal failure. Ideally, you should choose an event or experience that you have not yet talked about with others in detail or that you are hesitant to disclose. Remember, no one will see this but you.

Step 3: Express your deepest emotional concern

It is extremely important that you really speak from the heart and delve into your deepest thoughts and feelings. Write down whatever comes to mind, but be sure to describe your feelings and emotions.

Step 4: Stop writing at the end of twenty minutes

Put your writing away in a private and confidential place.

Step 5: Do the exercise twice more

Write about the same experience all three times. Your writing exercises should be separated by several days to a week.

Step 6: Read your writing aloud

After the final writing exercise, privately read aloud what you have written. Are there any areas where you need help and guidance in placing this event in a realistic context and learning from it for the future? Write them in your journal or in the space below.

If you believe that you have already been able to read your narrative aloud with lessened emotional reactivity, write down what you think you learned from this event.

How will this new information or understanding about the event help you to be less distressed or more patient with yourself in the future? For example, you may find that you are more likely to accept other people's faults, or you may become more patient with your initial emotional reactions to upsetting events, realizing that having feelings is a normal part of life.

_____

_____

_____

_____

_____

_____

_____

Step 7: Evaluate your progress

Do you feel more patient with yourself now about your emotional response to the painful and traumatic moments in your life? If you found this technique helpful, follow the same steps anytime you find yourself fearful to think about an upsetting experience or feel impatient about your own emotional distress in reaction to an upsetting event.

There is a consensus among psychologists and physicians that the experience of negative emotions is a basic part of every person's life. Rather than try to take the time to understand negative feelings and work toward finding ways to better manage them, many people try to cover up, ignore, or suppress negative emotions when they occur. The suppression of feelings can have very serious consequences for your heart as well as other bodily systems. On the other hand, when you speak or write from your heart and express the emotions that are part of the difficult times in your life, you make an important first step toward caring for yourself and restoring your health.

9

Emotional Tool:
Fostering Acceptance

Too often, self-help books focus on ways to reduce negative emotions such as depression, anxiety, or anger without addressing ways to increase positive emotions such as acceptance. You may be wondering how learning to foster acceptance can improve your overall health. Although we could spend most of this chapter explaining the ways scientists explain how this may work on a physical level, the simple answer is that when you learn to accept yourself and others, you don't have to spend so much of your mental, physical, and emotional energy trying to avoid or escape negative feelings. Through the practice of acceptance, you are able to value both the positive and negative aspects of being alive and to increase your wisdom. With regard to heart disease, Carels and colleagues (2004) recently found that among a group of patients with heart failure, those who were more accepting of their illness and other life stressors experienced fewer physical symptoms (for example, chest pain and heaviness, shortness of breath) as compared to those who tended to avoid thinking about their troubles.

ACCEPTANCE VS. AVOIDANCE

Some people have difficulty seeing that disappointment, loss, pain, and suffering are a normal part of life. These experiences occur for everyone, even those individuals who manage to live full and rewarding lives. Despite this fact, many people exert far too much energy avoiding such experiences. Such avoidance can often extract a heavy cost. With regard to heart disease, for example, the general tendency to cope with problems by avoiding them has been found to increase mortality risk among patients with congestive heart failure (Murberg, Furze, and Bru 2004). We're not suggesting that you seek out ways to experience loss, disappointment, or pain. However, many therapists support the idea that through acceptance of the inevitability of life's negative experiences, you are likely to stop trying to find ways to avoid them.

HOW AVOIDANCE SETS YOU UP FOR FAILURE

When you try to control or deny your emotions, it is as if you expect yourself to be immune to feelings. Since no human being can escape emotions, you are setting yourself up to fail—you can never avoid the unavoidable. In addition, people frequently allow the experience of negative emotions to block out any positive experiences, based on the faulty expectation or assumption that the full range of both positive and negative human experiences cannot exist at the same time. Think about your own attempts to control or avoid negative feelings. Very often, such efforts don't work very well, actually make you feel worse, and even antagonize other people in your life because of the barriers you place between yourself and them. Some of our heart patients are surprised to learn that increasing their acceptance of life's stressors can be a key to unlocking many of their difficulties. When they learn a different approach, allowing themselves to have positive experiences despite the presence of negative feelings and the presence of heart disease, they find that they can actually decrease the distress over time.

WHY ACCEPTANCE IS GOOD FOR YOUR WELL-BEING

None of us are strangers to suffering, whether through medical illness, interpersonal arguments, difficulty making changes, stressful jobs, loss of loved ones, destructive family experiences, or social injustice. This is all part of the human experience, just as are close personal ties, moments of laughter, spiritual or intellectual insights, achievements, and joyous celebrations. Problems and distressful emotions are part of the human experience. The presence of pain, frustration, or sadness should not be viewed as being equal to depression, resentment, or hopelessness. It's the avoidance—that is, not accepting your feelings—that can often lead to clinical symptoms of distress.

ACCEPTING LIFE'S NEGATIVES

Accepting (rather than avoiding) the inevitable pain and suffering of life can serve as a powerful way to break free of the desire to control yourself and others. It can also help to increase your ability to cope with such suffering. We have seen many patients enter therapy with the faulty belief that if they could just get rid of the bad feelings they are experiencing, then they would have a better life. Indeed, distressing thoughts, feelings, and memories are often the reason why people seek therapy. However, many people don't realize that mental health is associated more with managing uncomfortable feelings effectively than with getting rid of them.

Many people also believe that their negative thinking and upsetting emotions are evidence of their own weaknesses, disease, laziness, or uniquely unfortunate circumstances. However, these beliefs are typically based upon faulty rules or logic in the form of self-talk that people have inadvertently learned from parents, peers, and their culture. Below are some examples of destructive messages you may have heard from others regarding emotions while you were growing up.

> *You have to get over your bad feelings and stop whining about things.*
> *Happy people don't get upset.*
> *It's silly (or stupid) to have these feelings.*
> *Stop crying! For goodness' sake, control yourself!*
> *You have no reason to be angry.*
> *What do you mean you're afraid? There's nothing to be afraid of.*

If you heard similar messages when you were younger, then you, like many people, have learned to be critical of your feelings, or embarrassed or frightened by them. Rather than view them as a normal and helpful part of being human, you have come to view them as evidence of being weak, crazy, out of control, or unhappy, or even as punishment from God. In order to learn to cope more effectively with the stresses and problems of everyday life, you'll need to make a major shift in attitude toward acceptance.

SHIFT YOUR ATTITUDE TO ONE OF ACCEPTANCE

Shifting your attitude to one of acceptance involves relinquishing control or letting go of the inner critic who tells you that you must deny or minimize all emotional suffering. Instead, you can use your experience as a guide to help you discover how to better manage your feelings and alter any ineffective patterns of behavior that result from your tendencies to avoid or fight off your feelings.

Psychologist Steven Hayes and his colleagues have developed a type of psychotherapy referred to as *acceptance and commitment therapy* (1999). Through this counseling approach, people learn to recognize when they engage in an ongoing, self-defeating, and unworkable internal dialogue in order to avoid emotional distress. One important idea that people learn through this treatment is that this struggle to avoid feelings is in their own mind. By cultivating acceptance, many people have come to learn that they can let go of this hopeless inner struggle and abide the presence of difficult situations or negative feelings, even if they are not sure what to do about them.

Think about your own current struggles. Our patients who are having difficulty with acceptance often say things like, "I know I shouldn't let this bother me," "This is a stupid way to feel," and "I hate feeling this way." In fact, many people we have counseled over the years believe that a "good" life is based upon being emotionally stronger, getting greater approval, controlling other people's reactions, achieving more power, having the most fun, gaining more recognition, or being taken care of. We call these *feeling fables* because they are stories or folktales about feelings, similar to fairy tales. Although they are not true, they often pass as such from one generation to the next. When you hear these fables from a very young age, you learn to say these things repeatedly to yourself, and as a result, you actually start to believe them. Inherent in so many of these feeling fables is the belief that negative feelings can and should be controlled, eliminated, or wiped out. When people become extremely depressed and hopeless, they may even resort to self-harm or suicide just to get rid of such bad feelings.

STOP BELIEVING IN FEELING FABLES

Get ready to stop believing in your feeling fables and let go of your need to control your emotions. Because you are not a robot, you can't control your feelings—you can only control how you react or behave when you experience them. With the tool provided below, we will help you learn to give up your personal feeling fables and accept negative emotions as simply part of being human. You'll learn to accept that there are situations over which you have little control.

PRACTICING ACCEPTANCE

As you follow the steps below, remember that when you accept problems, distress, and painful emotions as inevitable for everyone, you'll realize that your self-worth and goals for a purposeful and meaningful life are not equal to a perfectly happy or pain-free existence. This can free you to learn from challenges or heartache and make effective decisions about what is important to you or what you want to change. As you allow and accept negative emotions as simply a part of your human experience, you can become more willing to see how feelings can serve as a useful tool to help you understand yourself and solve difficult life problems.

Take out your notebook or journal in order to record your entries. Be sure to label them properly so you can locate this exercise later.

Step 1: Write down a current situation that is difficult to accept

Be sure to describe the situation as clearly or objectively as possible. Does this situation involve limitations related to your heart problems? Are you having difficulty accepting that you are getting older? Have your children or spouse changed in any significant way? Write down any situation that is currently difficult for you to accept. It is likely that you have strong feelings associated with this situation. Move on to the next step to identify the feelings you are experiencing.

Step 2: Write down your feelings about the situation

From the list provided below, check off the feelings you have about this situation, particularly feelings that make this situation distressful or those feelings that you most wish to avoid or have difficulty admitting you have.

- ☐   fear

- ☐   sadness

- ☐   anger

Step 3: Write down the thoughts or concerns that specifically pertain to these feelings

Now that you have identified the problem situation and associated feelings, you are ready to describe your concerns or thoughts about experiencing the distressing emotions that you are trying to avoid.

Step 4: Identify your personal feeling fables

Review your answer to step 3 and see if you can identify, in the descriptions of your thoughts, the presence of any of the following feeling fables. Check off any that apply to you.

- ☐   *It is important to get rid of bad feelings immediately.*

- ☐   *People who are mentally healthy can control and eliminate bad feelings.*

- ☐   *Being well-adjusted psychologically means not having any bad feelings.*

- ☐   *If I am sad, frightened, or angry, I must be weak or stupid.*

- ☐   *Crying, sadness, or anger will always make matters worse.*

- ☐   *People who are in control of their lives are generally able to control how they react and feel.*

Step 5: Get real! Know the facts about feeling fables

This step will help you to begin to accept your own feelings and prepare you to complete step 6 with a greater acceptance of these emotions. Consider the facts related to each fable below and expose the feeling fable for what it is: pure fiction. Read carefully the actual facts that contradict each feeling fable, using your own knowledge and experience to confirm these facts.

Fable: It is important to get rid of bad feelings immediately.

Fact: This is simply not true. Negative thoughts, feelings, and memories can be very useful in helping you to notice things about your life that are meaningful to you or that need to change. When bad feelings occur, you are already hurting. It makes sense to care for yourself and try your best to manage your feelings so that you understand *why* you are hurting.

Fable: People who are mentally healthy can control and eliminate bad feelings.

Fact: People who are in control of their lives may be in control of their behavior, but they rarely need to try to control their feelings. This is an important distinction. For example, if you are treated unfairly, it is important not to ignore your feelings of sadness, disappointment, or anger. How you choose to act on those feelings, however, is in your control.

Fable: Being well-adjusted psychologically means not having any bad feelings.

Fact: Being well-adjusted and mentally healthy means being able to notice and manage negative feelings without the need to analyze or justify the feeling. Bad feelings are more likely to pass if you don't spend significant time trying to rationalize their existence. You do not ever have to blame someone else for your feelings. They are yours . . . they are present . . . accept them . . . period.

Fable: If I am sad, frightened, or angry, I must be weak or stupid.

Fact: When negative emotions are intense, it is common to experience tearfulness, crying, confusion, nervous energy, or agitation. After all, emotions are a very physical experience. You may experience physical sensations, or your concentration may be interrupted. Expressing difficult feelings can also create an energy drain and result in feelings of fatigue. These are all predictable emotional side effects. If you view negative emotions as an inevitable part of being alive and can tolerate such physical reactions in yourself and others, this is a strength, rather than a weakness.

Fable: Crying, sadness, or anger will always make matters worse.

Fact: It is a very common mistake to believe that the remedy to a difficult situation is to deny the negative feelings. This does not solve the problem. By acknowledging and accepting your feelings, you are able to concentrate on ways you may be able to manage your feelings effectively or change the situation for the better.

Fable: People who are in control of their lives are generally able to control how they react and feel.

Fact: Although people who are in control of their lives often understand why they experience an unpleasant or bad feeling, it is unrealistic to expect that such feelings can be eliminated by understanding alone. For example, if you are very sad because you have suffered a loss or you're angry over an injustice, it is easy to see that under-standing the trigger for these feelings does not make the feeling go away. Being psycho-logically healthy means being willing to experience a wide range of emotions. Being able to admit that you are not always happy, learning to have negative moments while recognizing that you can still live effectively, represents a true path to personal peace.

Step 6: Experience the feelings

Now that you are less likely to avoid your feelings, you can allow yourself to make a commitment and be willing to experience your feelings without judging yourself. Use the feelings to understand what is important to you. Rather than criticizing your feelings, take the stance of objective reporting, and write down what you learn about accepting feelings. Allow your attitude to shift from avoidance to interest and curiosity about your feelings. Let your negative feelings help you to understand the challenges in accepting the negative event, change, or loss you identified in step 1.

Step 7: Sign a personal contract to make a commitment

Sign in the space below in order to make a commitment.

I, _____ ,
make a firm commitment to consider my distressful feelings as part of being human. I understand that my feelings can help me to understand myself better, help me to accept change and loss as a part of life, and provide me with ways to improve my life and help others.

Step 8: Face the situation

Using your new commitment to accept your feelings, write a plan in your journal for how you will face the situation you identified in step 1 and foster acceptance of the situation. Some people begin their plan by choosing one fear that they will confront in order to take the first step.

Step 9: Note your progress

As you begin to carry out your plan, make sure to note your progress in your journal by indicating ways in which fostering acceptance has helped you with the following goals:

- understanding yourself better

- accepting change and loss as part of life

- improving your life and helping others

AN IMPORTANT POINT TO REMEMBER

As you practice the steps to acceptance, be willing to get up again! When people have trouble with acceptance, they often say that it is too difficult to do and that they doubt that they will ever accept certain negative events. It is almost as if they are saying that in order to accept something, they must agree with it and experience no negative feelings. This is an impossible task. No wonder so many people give up! Acceptance means that you tolerate your negative feelings and are willing to experience or see suffering as part of life—maybe even one that allows you to value the other experiences more intensely, the ones in which you don't have to suffer.

As you successfully work to accept the first situation, go ahead and use this same tool to address other events, changes, or losses you have difficulty accepting.

10

Emotional Tool: Learning to Forgive

Sustained anger, chronic hostility, and the inability to forgive those who have hurt you can all serve as major obstacles to sound heart health (Miller et al. 1996). Further, failure to forgive others can worsen symptoms of depression and anxiety that already exist. Forgiveness researchers Robert Enright and Richard Fitzgibbons (2000), for example, point out that people who have difficulty managing their depression are often additionally wrestling with feelings of anger over painful memories and life experiences. Moreover, fears of losing control and exploding in anger can create more stress. Taken all together, the evidence is compelling that an inability to forgive others can actually intensify anger, hostility, anxiety, and depression and can be "toxic" to your heart. The good news is that the reverse can also be true. For example, a recent study reported that people who were able to forgive in response to interpersonal conflict improved their cardiovascular reactivity to stress (Lawler et al. 2003).

Although some people initially think of forgiveness as an act of weakness or "backing down," the truth is that successfully learning to forgive can be a great strength, a gift you give yourself. This gift gives you the freedom to move on with your life with a greater sense of well-being and a lighter heart.

ARE YOU STRUGGLING WITH FORGIVENESS?

Learning how to forgive may seem to be a daunting and challenging task. We have found that the way people think about the act of forgiveness can actually be part of this difficulty. For example, you may have a desire for justice and believe that in order for you to be able to forgive people who disappointed, hurt, or injured you in some way, they must first understand what they have done wrong and "pay" for their actions. You may have learned to equate forgiveness with excusing, minimizing, rationalizing, or justifying the hurt. These views are actually inaccurate, and in fact they prevent you from using forgiveness as a way of transforming your suffering into a sense of inner strength.

There is an old saying, "The person who holds on to anger and seeks revenge should dig two graves." For people with heart problems, this saying can be especially true. Holding on to an unforgiving attitude can be toxic to your health and will block you from moving on with your life. When you consider that you have probably been hurt or injured in some way already, why not choose to do something healing for your heart by freeing yourself from the past hurts and current hostility?

COMMON OBSTACLES TO FORGIVENESS

Before we provide you with the tools to practice forgiveness in your own life, let's look at several common roadblocks to the path of forgiveness. Awareness of these roadblocks is the first key to overcoming them.

The Fear of Forgiving

There may be times when you want to forgive but find yourself getting stuck because you are afraid. In this case of "forgiveness fear," someone is asking you for forgiveness, but you find it very difficult to meet this request. You realize that this person may be sorry, but you have been hurt or let down and you are fearful to trust the person's apology and promise of change. We have seen this fear in people who want to forgive a partner for an extramarital affair, for example, but struggle with the expectation that by forgiving their spouse or partner, they must be able to trust the person again. It is important to remember that forgiveness does not equal trust. Practicing forgiveness simply means that you are willing to let go of your anger. Trust, on the other hand, occurs over time with repeated experiences in which you learn that you can count on the person to support you and treat you with respect. However, in order to begin to trust someone again, you first have to forgive. In order to forgive, you must be willing to face your fears.

People Who Are Not Sorry for Their Actions

In another situation, you may experience difficulty forgiving because the person who hurt you is not sorry or remorseful. In fact, such people may believe that they have done nothing wrong and may actually view you as the one at fault. In this case, you may find yourself trapped by the sense of injustice you experience in response to such people's selfishness and lack of insight. You may believe that it is important to convince such a person, as well as others, that some harm was inflicted. The obstacle here is that you see yourself as thwarted in your efforts to forgive until the other person acknowledges being wrong and having caused you pain. The assumption here is that you cannot begin to forgive until this person is able to see and appreciate your side of the matter. This is not true. You do not have to wait to be asked for forgiveness in order to start forgiving! Your ultimate concern should be about your health, not who's right or wrong.

START LEARNING TO FORGIVE TODAY

It is extremely important to remember that letting go of anger does not have to involve pretending that nothing happened or excusing the injury done by someone else. Forgiveness is not the same as pardoning, condoning, forgetting, or even reconciliation (Enright 2001). Although forgiveness works best when the other person is sorry, you can still forgive and at the same time decide not to invest time and energy trying to build a deeper relationship with individuals who are reluctant to take responsibility for their actions.

Think about people who were the victims of crimes and reported that they were able to forgive those who had hurt them. People who have experienced this type of forgiveness often also report that it is important to focus on their own healing, trying to understand their own experience of hurt, enhancing their own skills of empathy and compassion, and eventually letting go of their anger and resentment (but not denying these feelings). Such efforts enable you to move your life forward and can actually foster heart health (Witvliet, Ludwig, and Vander Laan 2001).

TOOLS FOR LEARNING FORGIVENESS

The tools described in the following sections will help you learn how to forgive. Remember that the inability to forgive can last longer—and therefore be more harmful to your health—than the original injury, insult, or injustice.

The first tool, a five-step plan for forgiveness, is designed to serve as a guide when you wish to forgive but are having difficulty getting started in putting your "change of heart" into action. We also provide advice about how you can use this plan if you are trying to forgive yourself.

The second tool, "The 30 Percent Solution," can be used to navigate the challenge of forgiving others who may be not sorry for their actions.

CREATING A CHANGE OF HEART: FORGIVING BY LETTING GO

Making forgiveness work to strengthen a relationship is a five-step process. When someone is asking you for forgiveness, and you have determined that you want to work on the relationship but you experience "forgiveness fears," the following five steps can increase the likelihood that another's request for forgiveness, plus your hard work at forgiving, will have positive results for you and your heart. You can remember these five steps with the acronym LET GO.

L – Listen.

E – Expect change.

T – Try a new plan.

G – Give away the anger.

O – Observe and notice change.

Step 1: Listen

Listen to the person asking for forgiveness. A true desire to repent and ask forgiveness indicates that the person understands he has done something that resulted in another person's pain or hurt. A person who is truly sorry or experiences regret is aware that his behavior—whether intentional or not—resulted in another person's suffering. Your ability to listen is important at this point, because you must try to see through the other person's eyes and truly hear what he is trying to say. If it is not clear to you that the person asking for forgiveness recognizes that his behavior resulted in pain or hurt, ask him directly if he understands this to be true. He should be able to recognize this. If you are trying to forgive yourself, this also holds true. You must be ready to accept that your actions or behavior caused someone else pain, whether or not that was your intention.

Step 2: Expect change

A person who is truly remorseful over what she has done will communicate a sense of certainty that she intends not to engage in the same behavior in the future. For example, the adolescent who apologizes for staying out several hours past curfew by sarcastically saying, "I'm sorry" is less likely to be asking for forgiveness compared to the one who understands the consequences of her behavior and indicates that she is serious about changing her behavior.

Although the person's actions resulted in unpleasant consequences for others, she would not have engaged in the behavior if there were not some personal benefit. Ask the person who is requesting forgiveness why she is certain that she will not engage in the same behavior in the future, when these actions held some benefit for her in the past. If she is sincerely asking for forgiveness, she will be clear that she does not want to choose the same path. If you are trying to forgive yourself, you must also be clear that your goal is to do something different. *Asking for forgiveness requires a commitment.*

Step 3: Try a new plan

A person who honestly requests your forgiveness is implying that he will behave differently the next time he is faced with a similar situation. Therefore, ask him to tell you how he will manage his behavior when faced with similar choices and situations in the future. In order to make the changes that follow his request for forgiveness, he will need to have both a commitment and an actual plan in place for future choices. If you are forgiving yourself, you must also have a plan for how you will change your behavior under similar circumstances.

Step 4: Give away your anger

Let go of your anger and forgive the person who is seeking forgiveness. Decide what you will say to yourself when you experience the fear of being vulnerable and the urge to get angry with the person based on her past misdeeds. Remind yourself that the person you are forgiving has made a commitment to change, and focus on the changes she has made. If you are forgiving yourself, commend yourself for your own commitment to change and let go of any negative self-judgment.

Step 5: Observe and notice change

Keep watch for any changes in behavior that indicate that the person who asked for forgiveness is doing something different. Show your appreciation when this occurs. If the person is not making changes and is likely to behave in ways that hurt you in the future, you may want to reconsider whether or not you wish to work hard at rebuilding this relationship. The most important thing to remember is that *your act of forgiving is not a gift you bestow on the other person but a gift you give to yourself.* However, by following the steps above and listening carefully to the person asking for forgiveness, you will have some estimate of how likely he is to engage in the same behavior again. This will help you make your choices about maintaining the relationship.

THE 30 PERCENT SOLUTION

Since you can't control how other people think and feel, this tool gives you a way to control how *you* think and feel by focusing on your part of the forgiveness equation. This tool can be especially useful when the other person is not actually seeking your forgiveness. The next time you find yourself angry for more than several days, experience difficulty forgiving another person, or feel ready to blame someone for the problems you experience in your life, remember that in any argument or negative situation between people, *how you think or behave is contributing at least 30 percent to your current distress.*

Even if you have been unfairly accused or badly treated, you have a choice in how you will react. Regardless of what has happened to you, your own reactions probably account for about 30 percent of your current emotional state and inability to forgive. Moreover, your choices about how you think and act with regard to this situation will affect not only how you currently feel but also whether such situations will occur in the future.

Let's consider Bill, a heart patient we know. Bill had problems with anger prior to receiving a new pacemaker and was having difficulty adjusting to the changes in his life. Recently, he decided to attend his company picnic. However, he harbored a grudge against one of his coworkers, Joe, because of wisecracks Joe had made about Bill's poor performance at a softball game a year ago, at the last company picnic. Although Joe had made an insensitive joke at Bill's expense, Bill's own worries about his declining athletic ability and his low self-esteem contributed to his vulnerability in reacting angrily to Joe's wisecracks.

We taught Bill to apply the 30 percent solution to his difficulty forgiving Joe. In doing so, he decided to focus more on the pleasant experiences in his life and on strengthening his self-esteem so that Joe's wisecracks would not hurt him in the future. As he worked toward these goals for personal change, Bill was able to let go of the anger he was holding toward Joe. As a result, Bill began to view Joe in a more accurate light: as one who makes fun of others as a way to get attention. Bill still didn't care much for Joe, but he was able to forgive Joe's insensitivity to the extent that it no longer took away from his enjoyment with other friends and coworkers at the picnic.

THE 30 PERCENT SOLUTION

Step 1: Summarize the situation

Take out your journal and write down the following:

- the name of the person whom you are having difficulty forgiving

■   a brief description of how this person hurt you, how long ago this incident occurred, how you were hurt, and this person's behavior toward you (including what they said aloud) that you are finding difficult to forgive

Step 2: Identify your 30 percent

Now use the 30 percent rule to list the behaviors, thoughts, or actions on *your* part that may have contributed to the problem (even just a little). This might be difficult because you may not want to accept any blame for what happened. It will help if you do not think of your own reactions as the reason the other person hurt you—just identify what thoughts, feelings, or actions on your part may have contributed to the situation in which you were hurt, even in a small way. List these now in your journal.

Next, decide which thoughts, feelings, and actions you would like to change for the future. For example, if you believe that someone else is taking advantage of you, do you ever unintentionally encourage this by not being assertive? Perhaps increased assertiveness is a goal for you. Perhaps someone lied to you about something important. Is there any possibility that you have made it difficult for people to be honest with you? One personal goal may be to increase your patience or your tolerance of other opinions.

Step 3: Make a plan to change

Make a goal for changing the behavior, and break down your own goal into small steps in order to construct a realistic plan of action. Remember that being willing to change something in yourself does not justify the other person's behavior! For example, if people have taken extreme advantage of your good nature, deciding to set clearer limits on what others demand of you is not the same as saying that they were right and you were wrong. This may help you to better understand how you can reduce the likelihood of similar hurts occurring in the future.

Bill's plan of action included telling himself that Joe's opinion of him was not very important. In fact, Bill realized that it is impossible to control anyone else's opinion. In addition, Bill reminded himself that people like Joe seem to wisecrack in order to feel good about themselves at others' expense. He found himself actually feeling sorry for Joe in this regard. Finally, Bill made a commitment to take better care of himself by focusing his energies on the people in his life whom he enjoyed being with and who provided him with good support.

In your journal, write the answers to the following two questions:

■   What do you want to change?

■   How will you change it?

Step 4: Reward yourself for your progress

Congratulate yourself for making even small steps toward your goal. Remind yourself that others often act for their own psychological survival, and the way in which you have been hurt by their actions is more about their own desperation than about their intention directed toward you.

Write down the following affirmation on a small card in order to carry it in your wallet or purse, or write it on a sticky note and post it on your desk or mirror.

I will let go of my anger. I will forgive. I will move forward with my life, with all my heart, for my heart.

Congratulate yourself on taking steps to improve your life, maintain a healthy heart, and reduce the impact of other people's hurtful actions.

It's important to remember that this technique is designed not to excuse the other person's behavior but to help you improve the quality of your own life. Forgiveness can significantly reduce the emotional pain you feel. You will find that as you take note of your progress and work to make personal changes, you are closer to whom you want to be. As a consequence, you will experience less and less of an urge to hold on to your anger.

In your journal, write about your progress toward personal change.

You now have a record of the process you went through to forgive someone. You can look back at your answers again whenever you have difficulty forgiving someone in the future.

FINDING TEACHERS IN UNLIKELY PLACES

Do you remember the teachers you had throughout your life whom you would describe as most effective, those to whom you can credit your most significant learning experiences? What do you remember about such experiences that made them so important and memorable? You may be surprised to learn that when you catch yourself blaming or getting angry with someone who seems to be your enemy, if you use the 30 percent solution, this person who caused you so much hurt may actually provide you with a valuable learning experience.

When people are asked to describe their most powerful learning experiences, they often talk about their interactions with an effective teacher. What would you say to the idea that the very same people whom you find difficult to forgive may actually be thought of as teachers? Here's how it works. Effective teachers provide an opportunity for learners to advance and realize their unique potential. Think about how learning to let go of your anger toward someone else can actually serve to move you forward. Good teachers can provide an opportunity for learners to accomplish things that they didn't even think were possible. Right now you may be thinking, *I could never forgive that person.* You may surprise yourself by applying the 30 percent rule, learning more about yourself, feeling stronger, then letting go of your anger.

Important learning experiences with effective teachers often involve a struggle, similar to the difficulties in learning a complex task. Forgiving someone is a struggle, but it can also be a learning experience. Moreover, the fact that you are struggling with forgiveness means that it is difficult but not that it is impossible.

Finally, in describing the experience of learning from memorable or effective teachers, many people describe the teacher as someone who provides the opportunity and guidance to apply what is learned in a practical way. This is a critical part of the learning experience. You struggle with how to apply this learning to your day-to-day experience.

When you apply the 30 percent solution, you can learn valuable lessons as you learn more about yourself and apply this new knowledge to improve your life. We suggest that the next time you face a conflict with someone whom you find difficult to forgive, try using the 30 percent solution by telling yourself that there may be a clear and purposeful reason you are presented with this person in this situation at this time in your life. Ask yourself, *What can I learn about myself?* Tell yourself, *This can be a valuable learning experience.*

FINAL THOUGHTS

Learning to forgive can be an especially important part of your plan for improving your heart health, and it may be one of the most challenging tools to put into practice. If you practice these tools and continue to have some difficulty learning to forgive, you may need a little extra help from some of the other chapters. For example, you can learn to change your inaccurate and unforgiving thoughts by trying the thinking tools (chapters 12 and 13). You may also find that the relaxation tools (chapters 14, 15, and 16) can help by teaching you how to quiet down your body from an angry state of arousal. We are confident that when these tools are applied together, anyone can successfully learn to forgive.

11

Behavioral Action Tool: Enhancing Positive Experiences

As you consider the title of this chapter, you may be thinking, *Enhancing positive experiences sounds pleasant enough, but what does this have to do with improving my heart health?* Put simply, it is good medicine for your heart to love, laugh, and experience pleasure. Research that we conducted years ago demonstrated the potential power of positive moments—like those found through laughter and humor—to reduce depressive reactions to stressful situations (Nezu, Nezu, and Blissett 1988). When you consider the destructive impact of negative states such as depression and anger on your heart, it is not surprising that subsequent research has strongly suggested positive emotional states can serve as an important tool in the prevention of heart disease (Pearsall 1998). When you are open to creating a greater number and variety of positive life activities, you not only experience a positive shift in your mood, but your body goes through physical changes that can be especially beneficial to your immune system and your heart (McCraty, Atkinson, and Tomasino 2003). On the other hand, when you have only a few pleasant activities, lack joyful experiences, or continue unproductive behavior, you feel depressed, stressed out, trapped, bored, and sad. Your body experiences strain and fatigue. When you have these feelings, it is common to put off or even avoid pleasant experiences. This can create a vicious cycle of depression by increasing feelings of sadness, irritability, or entrapment, leading to decreased motivation to do anything that brings you pleasure.

BREAKING FREE FROM THE VICIOUS CYCLE

What comes first? Do you feel depressed, fatigued, or irritable because you don't have enough pleasant events or experiences in your life, or do you fail to seek out and create such experiences because you are depressed or afraid? The answer is that it works both ways. The less you do for yourself, the more depressed and irritable you get, and the more depressed you get, the less you do.

The good news is that there are ways to change this downward spiral. There is a strong relationship between the positive experiences you create for yourself and your mood. In other words, by increasing pleasant experiences, you feel better. This approach to the treatment of depression was pioneered by psychologist Peter Lewinsohn and his colleagues (1978) and more recently augmented by others (Jacobson, Martell, and Dimidjian 2001). Such treatments, which are designed to help people experience more pleasant activities and reach personal goals, have been demonstrated in several scientific studies to be an effective way to manage and reduce negative moods such as depression. This approach works by teaching people how to overcome the tendency toward avoidance, withdrawal, and inactivity. If you have been feeling sad, distressed, irritable, or burned out, it is likely that your rate of pleasant activities (that is, big and small events that bring you a sense of enjoyment) is low. You are also probably not noticing pleasant experiences when they happen, not doing many of them, or not getting much pleasure from them when you do them. You may be wondering how to get yourself started or "activated." The steps of this tool will teach you how to

- make an inventory of your current level of activity

- make a list of the experiences and events you enjoy

- make a list of the experiences or positive events you want to increase (for example, ones you want to do more of, new ones you want to try)

- notice and enjoy the positive experiences you have

- get yourself activated in small steps to increase the frequency of pleasant activities

ENHANCING POSITIVE EXPERIENCES

Sometimes the effects of using this tool can be immediate, so let's get you started by helping you to make an inventory of your current activity level. This will give you a bird's-eye view of your activities over a week. Next, you will identify what activities are most important for *you*, rather than what other people think is enjoyable. This is an important point. When you think of activities that you wish you could do more often, your choices may be very different from those of other people. One person might enjoy going to the opera or socializing, while another prefers staying at home and reading a good book. One person might prefer to take the dog for a walk, while others would find it more pleasant to stay indoors and take a bath. Only when you focus on *your* life and what brings *you* pleasure will this tool have an effect on *your* mood.

Step 1: Make an inventory of your current activity level

First, make an inventory or log of your current level of activity as well as the current level of positive events that you experience. Using the daily activity inventory, keep track of what you are actually doing over a period of several days, entering in the activities that you engage in during each time period. For example, between 6:00 and 8:00 A.M., one patient, Jim, wrote down that he showered, dressed, watched morning news on TV, walked his dog, took vitamins, filled a coffee thermos, and answered some e-mail before leaving the house for work. Next, circle any activities that you view as pleasant. Jim circled "walked the dog."

It is important to complete the activity log over several days so that you have a good view of your activities over the week. For instance, you are likely to have a different schedule of activities or routines on workdays than on weekends or holidays. Copy these columns in your journal in order to have enough space to complete the activities log for an entire week.

Next, use the "Comments" column to indicate how you wish to change any of your daily routines. In other words, consider the activities you want to increase and the activities you want to decrease. Jim indicated that he wished he had time to enjoy a sit-down breakfast and read the morning newspaper. It was interesting to see that Jim's weekend activity log also did not include breakfast. He reported feeling overwhelmed that he had all of his weekend errands and chores on his mind, and he usually tries to get started on these activities early. However, none of the errands and chores were marked off as pleasant. Jim was not using his weekend time to do more of what he wanted to do. As a consequence, he lost the opportunity to feel better.

Next, place a check mark next to any time period where you indicated that you have no pleasant activities occurring. If you have many pleasant activities occurring in every time period, it is likely you do not need to complete this exercise, because you are already making sure that you have a full range of positive experiences in your life.

Activities Inventory		
Waking Hours	**Activities** (Circle those that are pleasurable.)	**Comments** (Indicate how any time periods could be made more pleasurable.)
6:00–8:00 A.M.		
8:00–10:00 A.M.		
10:00 A.M.–noon		
noon–2:00 P.M.		
2:00–4:00 P.M.		
4:00–6:00 P.M.		
6:00–8:00 P.M.		
8:00–10:00 P.M.		
10:00 P.M.–midnight		

You will use this inventory later to replace an unpleasant activity with a pleasant one or to add more pleasant activities to your schedule. But first, you need to decide what is pleasant for you.

Step 2: Make a list of experiences and events you enjoy

Plan on taking about thirty minutes to an hour to write down in your journal all the events, activities, experiences, and people in your life that you experience as pleasant. You should schedule an uninterrupted block of time when you can concentrate on doing this task. At the end of this chapter, we provide sample lists of positive experiences that other people have identified. This may help you to create your own list, but remember to write down in your journal only the things that truly apply to you.

Although people differ regarding what experiences they find pleasant or joyful, there are a number of activities that psychologists, such as Peter Lewinsohn (1978), have referred to as "mood-related activities" because they are strongly associated with how you feel. These activities are often divided into three categories: social activities, personal accomplishments, and feel-good activities.

Social activities. These are activities through which you experience feeling respected, understood, valued, needed, supported, and loved by others. Some examples include being with someone who cares about how you feel, telling a joke, working on a project with a friend, caring for a child, and being asked your opinion.

Accomplishments. These are activities that give you a sense of achievement, satisfaction, individuality, success, or independence. Some examples include finishing a term paper, building a bookcase, writing a clever e-mail, reading a book, or cooking a good meal. One patient we know felt a good sense of reward after she cleaned windows!

Feel-good activities. These are activities or experiences that simply feel good and contribute to the joys of living. These include smelling baked bread, sweating during exercise, slipping into a hot tub, getting a back rub, watching a candle glow in a darkened room, or smelling the salty air at the seashore.

Step 3: Target experiences or positive events to increase

Look over the list you developed in step 2. These are all opportunities to increase your pleasant experiences. Circle the ones you most want to prioritize, even if you are not exactly sure how you will work them into your schedule or routine. Prioritize those activities that are most important, most pleasant, or even most feasible for you to work on during the coming weeks and months.

Step 4: Make yourself aware; notice positive experiences

Now go over your list and underline those positive activities that you actually did and experienced as joyful or pleasant. For example, suppose you wrote down "talk to my children," and you actually had the opportunity to visit with your son or daughter or play with your grandchild last week. If you were able to enjoy this experience at the time, then underline it.

Now go back over the list once again and place an X next to the items that you actually experienced but failed to be mindful of, take in fully, or enjoy. For example, maybe you took a nice hot shower, an experience that you usually find pleasant, but you were worried about something at work and you failed to stop and be aware, or mindful, of the experience. Instead, you hardly noticed the shower and spent the entire time lost in negative thinking. If so, then you missed out on a pleasurable activity.

Next, determine your activity score. Add up the total number of items that you wrote down. Now subtract the number of items that you underlined. This is your pleasant activities score. How many of your possible pleasant items are you currently experiencing? If your score is twice the number that you underlined, it's time to get yourself activated to increase pleasant activities.

Finally, look at the number of items marked with an X. These are experiences that you are missing out on because you are not fully attentive to them. It is time to discover the pleasant events that are already part of your life right now!

Step 5: Make a plan to get activated.

Look over the entire list one more time and pick one item that you circled or targeted as a priority—something you find pleasant and would like to do more often. This may not be easy, because it may require some shifting of time and responsibilities. However, now is the time to revisit your activity inventory to help you discover where you could add this new activity.

Find an activity period where there are currently no pleasant activities listed and where you would be willing to make some small but significant changes. For example, Jim decided that he wanted to make changes in his weekday routine such that he could enjoy a sit-down breakfast at least once in a while. Looking over his inventory, he realized that he could get the newspaper delivered to his doorstep and read the news-paper (an activity he enjoyed) rather than watch the television news (an activity he did not particularly enjoy). He also noticed that he had some time in the evening to complete his e-mail correspondence, after dinner. This allowed him the time in the morning to have a sit-down breakfast and read the newspaper. He reported that he felt less rushed and more able to enjoy breakfast. In addition, he said that choosing differ-ent microwave breakfast items and anticipating the different breakfasts he would have during the week made his shopping trips more pleasant.

Now look at the items marked X. Again, these are the activities that you actually experienced but failed to notice, take in, or enjoy. These are happening already, but you are not getting the full benefit of the positive effects they can have on your physical well-being. Choose three items that you will make a commitment to notice and take in (for example, your baby's smile, the friendly salesperson at the store, singing along with your favorite music, lighting a candle at Shabbat, hugging your friend). Write them down now.

Make a commitment to add one new activity (or change a routine by replacing an old activity with a new one) and notice three activities that are already happening each week.

Next, pick a time each week when you will take a few moments to rate yourself on a scale of 1 to 10 (1 being the lowest and 10 being the highest) regarding two questions:

■   What is your overall level of pleasant events or positive experiences?

■   What is your overall mood?

These ratings are not meant to be a rating of your emotions at any one specific time during the week. For example, in a given week, you may have cried because you missed a friend, had several new joyful experiences, become frustrated in traffic, or started to feel sick due to an impending cold. You may have been able to enjoy eating a good meal or helping a friend, but perhaps you became preoccupied with angry or aggressive thoughts during a disagreement with your spouse or partner. Each of these events, taken as a snapshot, would yield a different rating. However, looking over the week in general, how would your rate your mood?

Monitor the direction and stability of your mood ratings over several weeks. If you increase the quality of your mood, there's a good chance that your commitment to increasing pleasant events is having an effect.

If your mood is not improving, continue to add one more activity each week to your list, and be sure to actually do the activities. Also look at the activities that you marked with an X, and take the time to enjoy them more. Allow yourself a few extra moments to notice how pleasant the experience is. Focus your attention and be mindful of your delight in the experience. We remember one of our patients, Joan, who reported that she had laughed very little over the past few months. When she made it a goal to be mindful of others and smile more often, she realized how many people were actually smiling at her. Before, she had failed to notice and take pleasure in this simple human connection because she had been focused on worrying about the past, over which she no longer had control.

It is important to remember that no matter how disconnected, depressed, or hopeless you feel, there are always some activities and thoughts that are pleasant, even for a fleeting moment. If you find yourself saying that you are too busy, too burned out, or too undeserving to systematically change your routine and weekly activities to give yourself more pleasant experiences, then this tool is precisely what you need to help activate yourself!

Positive Experiences

Social Activities		
being with friends	going to a party	going to a sports event
going to a convention	meeting someone new	playing with children
being helped with something	going to a church, temple, shrine, or mosque	going to a music concert, ballet, or theater production
having an honest conversation	being with people with similar interests	going to a fair, carnival, or zoo
discussing something interesting	going to a race (horse, car, or boat)	going walking, hiking, or camping
having lunch with someone you like	planning or organizing an event	having a friend come to visit

Social Activities		
seeing good things happen to your family or friends	talking to your children or grandchildren	talking to someone in an Internet chat room
talking about philosophy, morals, or religion	playing cards or board games	playing tennis, golf, or another sport
dating	talking on the telephone	going to a reunion
going to the movies	kissing or hugging	giving gifts
being at a wedding, bar mitzvah, baptism, graduation, or birthday party	having a cup of coffee, cup of tea, cocktail, glass of wine, or beer with someone	visiting someone in a hospital, rehab facility, or prison
going to school or class	loaning something	giving a party
getting letters or cards	helping someone	coaching someone
introducing people to each other	going to an outdoor event	buying something for your family
sending letters, cards, or notes	being told that you are needed	being at a family get-together
being invited out	visiting friends	having sexual relations
having someone agree with you	talking about hobbies or interests	finding out about someone's joy or sorrow
watching attractive men or women	giving a massage or back rub	expressing your love to someone
smiling at people	being counseled	seeing old friends
going to an auction or sale	expressing your appreciation to someone	doing things with children
talking to people at work	doing volunteer work	being complimented
hearing a good sermon or speech		

Accomplishments		
playing a sport	hiking or climbing	doing artwork
making a contribution to a charity organization	being prepared for a test or job	planning a trip or vacation
going to a lecture	driving skillfully	singing
redecorating your room or home	working on cars or machines	working on your computer
boating	restoring antiques	preparing special food
completing a difficult task	solving a problem or puzzle	writing a story, poem, novel, or play
writing a note	cooking	skiing
exploring unknown places	speaking a foreign language	playing a musical instrument
working at your job	losing weight	having an original idea
solving a personal problem	making food or crafts to give away	bowling or playing pool or billiards
gardening or landscaping	learning a new skill	competing at sports
taking photographs	reading a map	washing clothes
giving a speech or lecture	writing a letter, paper, or essay	getting a job advancement
hearing a joke	making a major purchase	winning a bet
eating a good meal	hunting	horseback riding
doing a project in your own way	doing heavy outdoor work	completing a crossword puzzle
fishing	reading a paper	swimming
playing catch	having a debate	doing needlework
making people laugh	starting a new project	building a fire
teaching someone	using your strength	receiving money
running, jogging, or walking	defending or protecting someone	waterskiing, surfing, or scuba diving
winning a competition		

Feel-Good Activities

being in the country	getting dressed up	watching the ocean
buying or picking flowers for yourself	buying something for yourself	reading spiritual or religious writings
giving something away	being at the beach	watching TV
reading stories, novels, poems, or plays	thinking about something good in the future	giving your opinion or advice
laughing	hugging	shaving
taking a shower or bath	taking a long car trip	riding in an airplane
being with an animal or pet	lighting or watching candles	combing or brushing your hair
praying or meditating	holding a baby	being in a sporty car
crying	taking a nap	wearing casual clothes
watching someone you love	looking at the stars or moon	listening to records or the radio
driving fast	singing to yourself	being in a city
putting on makeup	watching an animal	wearing new clothes
dancing	sitting in the sun	riding a motorcycle
sitting and being mindful	gambling	getting a massage
listening to nature sounds	thinking about people you like	feeling the presence of spiritual forces
getting ice cream	kicking leaves	having daydreams
making popcorn	being alone	renting a video
getting up early	going to a restaurant	washing your hair
getting up late	reminiscing	writing in a diary
practicing yoga	sleeping soundly	going to a hair salon
reading magazines	bird-watching	beachcombing
sitting in a café	going to a museum	eating snacks
noticing that you smell good	going to a library or bookstore	going to a health club or spa
going to a concert		

12

Thinking Tool: Changing Negative Thinking

Negative thinking habits are patterns of self-destructive thoughts that can lead to strong and distressing emotional reactions. If you have developed such negative thinking habits (and to some degree, most people do), it may be important to first understand how you have learned to think this way and what you can do to "unlearn" these thoughts. Continuous negative thinking can trigger negative emotions, which can then lead to harmful effects on your heart health.

WHERE HEART AND MIND MEET

In order to better understand how your heart and mind are connected, imagine that four different people are about to attend a meeting at work. The situation for all four people is the same: each person is planning a business event for the company and is required to give a progress report. They have all had some very good ideas about how to plan the event, but each has slightly underestimated the time or cost involved. Read each of the following four thoughts and see if you can identify the anxious thought (A), the depressive thought (D), the angry/hostile thought (H), and the realistically optimistic thought (O).

I hope I don't sound like a jerk. I get so scared when I have to talk in front of people.

I don't want to go to work today. I can't meet all those deadlines. I'm failing at this job.

These people don't appreciate how hard I work. What idiots! I can't stand their stupid faces.

I'm eager to share my current plans and get other people's opinions on how to trouble-shoot some of the problems with time and cost constraints.

If you labeled the thoughts A, D, H, and O (in that order), then you correctly identified each thought. Now imagine how each person feels upon walking into the meeting. You can easily see how each person's thinking is associated with a corresponding emotion. Finally, consider the accuracy of each person's thoughts. Objectively, the person with the realistic and optimistic set of thoughts is probably the most accurate. The other thoughts actually reflect negative thinking patterns that are exaggerated, overgeneralized, and basically incorrect. People learn to say such things internally, and although such thoughts are inaccurate, people believe them to be true because they occur automatically in response to stressful situations.

How you perceive and interpret various life events largely determines your consequent emotional and physical reactions. If your interpretation is negative (for example, fearful, angry, hostile, sad, worried, or hopeless), then your resulting emotional reaction is also likely to be negative. Conversely, if your interpretation is more positive and realistic, then the emotional reaction is more likely to be positive and realistic. Moreover, your interpretation can have a positive impact on your heart health. For example, the effects of a realistic and optimistic way of thinking have been found to be associated with a faster rate of physical and psychological recovery in a study of middle-aged men who underwent coronary artery bypass surgery (Scheier et al. 2003).

An important point to remember is that all negative thinking habits distort the truth, lack accuracy, and can negatively affect cardiovascular functioning. Therefore, the tool that we offer in this chapter will not teach you to simply say positive things to yourself. Rather, it will help you to make your thinking more accurate. We'll examine how each negative thinking habit distorts reality and why people may learn to make such critical or "heartbreaking" statements to themselves.

THOUGHTS THAT "BREAK YOUR HEART"

In previous chapters, we discussed how anxiety, anger, and depression are harmful to your heart. It will come as no surprise that the three types of thinking habits that are particularly "cardiotoxic," or potentially poisonous to your heart, are fearful thoughts, hostile thoughts, and depressive thoughts. These thoughts are so destructive to your psychological, emotional, and physical health that they have been associated, either individually or in combination, with heart disease (Sirois and Burg 2003) as well as many psychological or medical problems, including aggression, assault, murder, suicide, disorders of immune functioning, pain syndromes, substance abuse, and conflicts between couples, families, communities, and countries (Nezu, Nezu, and Lombardo

2004). Learning to make your thinking more accurate can be a very important tool for reducing your own negative thinking patterns and the likelihood of subsequent harmful health effects. Let's begin by learning more about these three different types of negative thinking patterns.

Fearful Thinking

When you are caught in a fearful or anxious thinking pattern, you become a prisoner to all that you fear. Because you are engaged in fearful thinking, much of your energy is focused on avoiding the unpleasant aspects of anxiety. This results in a continual preoccupation with your fears rather than the moments of your life. It is as if you decided to take a vacation that was focused on avoiding any discomfort rather than on experiencing the trip itself. If you've ever traveled, you know that in order to get the most out of the experience, you must be willing to do something different, experience some unfamiliar territory, and navigate the obstacles that occur along the way. In fact, for many people, these elements are the very reasons a vacation can be exciting! Fearful thinking, on the other hand, represents a constant attempt to keep things the same, avoid all uneasiness, and continually control your environment in order to feel safe.

Many people wonder how they have come to think this way. Learning can be a very complicated and often subtle process. First, you may have a temperament or predisposition to react in a specific physical manner more strongly or quickly than other people. In other words, the unpleasantness or discomfort you feel when afraid may cause more physical reactivity than it would for someone else. Another reason you might have such negative thinking habits may be that your parents, caregivers, siblings, peers, or other influential people have communicated—either intentionally or unintentionally—that emotional and physical distress are intolerable or represent something terrible. You learned that the experience of fear itself is something to avoid. Perhaps you can recall times when you were "afraid of being afraid." In most cases, people learn fearful thinking habits and avoidance due to a combination of these factors.

In addition, human brains appear to be structured or hardwired to learn to fear, because avoiding truly life-threatening events is important for survival. As human beings, we have a very well-tuned brain network to help us avoid true danger. Think about how quickly you react to a car coming toward you at a busy intersection or to a snake or flying insect while walking in the woods. The problem is that through many different types of conditioning or learning processes, people have learned to respond to many non-life-threatening situations, thoughts, and experiences as if they were very dangerous. For example, the dangers of failure, humiliation, embarrassment, or even negative feelings are circumstances that people learn to avoid as if their lives depended on it. The irony is that fearful and avoidant thinking and chronic anxiety can be far more threatening to your health than the inevitable failures, embarrassment, or short-lived negative reactions to bad events that are all simply a normal part of the human experience.

Recognizing Fearful Thoughts

In order to change your fearful thoughts, you will have to be able to recognize them or catch yourself making fear-based statements silently to yourself. Fear-based thoughts usually contain an anticipation of harm. Examples include when you hear yourself making internal statements that you may fail at something important or that other people may get angry with you. Your mind reasons that since you don't have total control over preventing something bad from happening, it is better to avoid it. Unfortunately, trying to avoid such anxiety-provoking thoughts only increases the likelihood that they will occur more frequently and intensely. For example, try not to think of the word "banana" for the next three minutes. If you are like most people, you are thinking right now, *How can I stop thinking of the word "banana"?* thus ensuring that you will constantly be thinking of that very word.

Another common fearful thought involves *mind reading,* or assuming that you know what others think when you have little or no proof. Examples of such fearful thoughts include *He thinks I'm crazy, They're probably laughing at me, I'm going to screw up,* or *She doesn't care about me.* Have you ever experienced any of these thoughts? In this case, your mind has decided to accept the worst possible outcome without any evidence rather than hope for the best and accept that you may have to endure some disappointment.

Often, people focus on the worst-possible scenario—for example, the likelihood that a plane is going to crash. Statistics prove that it is more likely that a person will get injured or die in a car accident than in a plane crash. Yet, some people focus on the worst-case scenario, allowing the horrors of a plane crash to "justify" their fear of flying but fearlessly getting into a car to travel. In this way, fear-based thinking is not only inaccurate, it is usually irrational.

When you engage in fearful thinking, you make the decision that the transient experiences of distress we all experience from time to time are terrible and catastrophic and must be avoided at all costs. Sometimes people with anxious thoughts believe that they are the only people who ever have them. However, that is particularly inaccurate; in fact, we all survive painful, embarrassing, or distressing thoughts and feelings in some way, every day.

Angry, Hostile, and Cynical Thoughts

It may sound like a paradox, because most of us don't think of hostile and angry people as scared or anxious, but angry, hostile, and cynical thoughts are actually quite similar to fearful thoughts. Consider a hostile or overbearing person who intimidates others. This individual has learned to intentionally stack the deck so the other person will always get the criticism, disapproval, or abuse. However, this is but another way to avoid any unpleasant experiences of failure, imperfection, or lack of control.

The difference between hostile thoughts and fearful thoughts is the content. Specifically, the content of hostile thoughts involves other people, those whom you can blame for your disappointments. You might view others, particularly those who disagree with you, as foolish and lacking intelligence or insight. When you engage in hostile thinking, your mind tells you that others don't respect you or recognize how important, smart, or great you are. You have learned that by seeing others as stupid, faulty, or unappreciative, you can avoid looking at any faults or problems of your own. Focusing on yourself may be too threatening and likely to engender very unpleasant emotions, so you have learned that it is better to engage in hostile thinking, keep such emotions away, and perceive yourself as in control. The problem is that you are likely to feel irritable and impatient with others most of the time. Unfortunately, it is you and your heart that will actually suffer.

Although people who have hostile thinking habits are less likely to see a counselor and seek help in changing (since they believe everyone else is at fault), many eventually do because they have experienced a personal, legal, financial, or medical setback that revealed their angry thinking or behavior as problematic. Because of the association between hostile thinking and medical conditions such as hypertension and cardiac arrhythmias, many heart patients are referred by their physicians to psychologists and counselors for help in changing their hostile thinking. Perhaps one of these situations applies to you.

You may be asking yourself how people learn to think in an angry or hostile way. If you have a tendency toward hostile thoughts, perhaps you were rewarded for being strong, independent, or tough during your childhood. Thinking of yourself in that way helped you to avoid being hurt. In this case, angry and hostile thinking represent another way to avoid fear and insecurity. Perhaps you were punished harshly for minor faults or mistakes and learned to tell yourself that such flaws are unacceptable and should be punished in others. Perhaps you were spoiled by your parents and they could not bear to see you upset, so you had to always find a reason why you should not or could not accept responsibility for periodic problems and distress that are experienced by all human beings.

As you can see, there are several ways that people learn to think in a hostile manner. We realize that admitting to yourself that you might have such thoughts is somewhat scary. Often, when we provide feedback to heart patients that they appear to be angry, perhaps because they are saying things that are hostile and cynical in nature, they initially get very defensive. Look deep in your heart and try to be as honest as possible as you continue to read this section.

Identifying Hostile Thoughts

Hostile thoughts are easy to identify if you are attentive and want to learn how to catch yourself.

Name-calling. They often take the form of name-calling in your head—for example, *That idiot, You moron,* or *What a creep.* Your mind is making sure that all blame for any distress you feel goes squarely on the shoulders of the other person. That way, you don't have to work at recognizing your own faults or changing anything you do.

The personalization error. Another common hostile thought process is to interpret any disappointment as directed personally toward you. For example, if other people's actions disappoint you, you tend to assume that their behavior is a direct attempt to hurt or insult you. We refer to this error in thinking as *personalization.*

Two types of personalization errors occur along with hostile thinking. The first type involves a tendency to view the motivation for another person's actions in terms of the consequences for you. For example, if you are verbally bullied, you see the bully's aggressive action as an attack on your weakness (as opposed to an example of his poor self-control). If someone challenges your argument, you see it as her attempt to make you look bad rather than her curiosity or attempt to make her own opinion heard. This heightens your emotional reaction, because you see the other person's behavior as always directed toward you instead of considering the wide range of explanations for such behavior, many of which have little to do with you.

A second type of personalization is concerned with comparisons you make between yourself and the other person. You often find yourself thinking *I would never do that* or *That's the wrong way to look at the situation.* This makes you the judge of what people should and should not do. In either type of personalization, the way to change your thoughts is to shift the focus of your thinking away from the other person and toward changing your own reactions.

Hostile Anger vs. Healthy Anger

Most hostile thoughts serve to deflect awareness of your own personal failures, problems, or imperfections. The desire to have such complete control over the imperfections in your life is impossible, and the need to protect your value and human worth from any faults is unnecessary. None of us is perfect! This is why hostile thoughts are so inaccurate—they attempt to maintain your perception of yourself as flawless.

There are times when angry thoughts, without the hostility and cynicism, can be useful and even healthy. When the angry thoughts do not focus on attacking others or protecting your image of yourself as flawless, they can sometimes help you understand what is important to you. Consider the anger you experience when viewing a social injustice or experiencing a problem that needs to be solved. In these cases, the angry thoughts are usually short-lived and result in positive action rather than chronic irritability.

Depressive Thinking

Depressive thoughts can seem like the opposite of hostile thoughts. When you are absorbed in depressive thinking, your mind is telling you that you are defective, inferior, or worthless. You usually do not engage in many fearful or hostile thinking patterns, because you are convinced that the reason things are unlikely to work out or make you happy is that you are basically inadequate. While people who engage in hostile thinking believe that they can control hurt or personal insult by blaming other people or avoiding the situation, with depressive thinking you tell yourself that change is hopeless and convince yourself that nothing much will turn out well. You view your-self as likely to fail, envision that your vulnerabilities will be revealed, and predict that you won't experience much pleasure or enjoyment in your life.

Whereas fearful and hostile thinking provide people with a false sense of control over their lives, depressive thinking reinforces the idea that the person has little control. When people feel chronically and severely hopeless, they may view acts of self-destruction or suicide as their only way out. If you are having specific self-destruc-tive or suicidal thoughts, it is extremely important that you learn to recognize them as inaccurate and seek help from a professional to overcome such thoughts.

Identifying Depressive Thoughts

The inaccuracy of depressive thoughts often lies in their exaggerated, magnified, and overgeneralized nature. Your mind is finding a small and isolated grain of nega-tive truth and making it huge. It is as if you're looking at your problems under an electron microscope. Upsetting but ordinary life situations—getting reprimanded at work, receiving a failing grade on a test, experiencing a disagreement with a family member, gaining weight, or receiving criticism—are viewed by the depressive mind as catastrophic, terrible, devastating, enduring, and all-encompassing phenomena. We describe these common depressive thinking errors in more detail below.

The magnification error. When you look at objects through a microscope or magnify-ing glass, they appear much larger than they really are. This depressive thinking error occurs when you emphasize a statement, act, or situation to a point where it is way out of proportion with its actual importance. Small comments or disappointments are seen as global and all-encompassing, and can become reasons for shame or self-hatred.

The opposite view is one in which you minimize the positive aspects of your own or someone else's behavior as a way of maintaining your depressive thoughts. For exam-ple, when someone notices one of your positive qualities, you may have a tendency to discount it, or if someone attempts to care for or nurture you, you tell yourself that you don't deserve it. Deep down, you assume that if you remain sad or hopeless, you will not be disappointed. The logic you use to justify your tight grip on depression is that holding on to sadness somehow protects you from further disappointment. Actually, such thinking only serves to bathe you in cardiotoxic emotions. Depression is far more harmful to your physical health than feeling sad when sad things happen.

The all-or-nothing error. When people engage in all-or-nothing thinking, they see the world in absolute black-and-white terms. For example, you might say to yourself, *How can I be happy when* (fill in the blank). *It's impossible.* Do you have any all-or-nothing thoughts with regard to the day-to-day challenges you face with health, work, family, or relationships? If so, it is important to practice changing your thoughts to be less absolute and more accurate. For example, *I can't be happy after the heart attack* could be changed to *It is difficult for me to enjoy some of the activities I did before* or *I am going through some tough times right now. I may need some extra help or support.*

There is an important reason for changing such all-or-nothing internal statements. When you say to yourself that something is impossible, you cease trying. Why would any logical person try to do something that is impossible? Accurate statements of difficulty or struggle, on the other hand, often maintain your motivation to continue working to solve the problems you are facing.

The overgeneralization error. When you make the error of overgeneralized thinking, you reach a general conclusion based upon a single incident. This internal statement is often held on to as a fact for a very long time. For example, you might say to yourself, *I'll never forget what he said to me.* In our own work conducting therapy with people suffering from medical illnesses, past traumas, or difficult life circumstances, we are often asked, "Wouldn't anyone with such a problem be depressed?" The fact is that many people live full and rewarding lives in the face of challenge and adversity. Helen Keller, who grew up deaf and without speech, once said, "The world is full of problems—it is also full of overcoming them." It is important to remember that creating positive and fulfilling experiences in your life does not mean pretending that problems do not exist; it means valuing your life in spite of such difficulties.

Understandably, it's harder to recognize and change depressive thinking when you are facing truly frightening and challenging life situations. However, inaccurate and depressive thoughts are likely to work against your efforts to manage difficult life circumstances, rather than help in any way. It is at such times that accurate, realistic, and balanced thoughts can be most important to your quality of life.

LEARNING TO CONFRONT AND CHANGE NEGATIVE THINKING

Unless you confront your negative thinking, the habits you have learned will likely be repeated, and you will continue to trigger a cycle of distressful emotional reactions. Negative thoughts can be changed. Through techniques of cognitive therapy pioneered by psychiatrist Aaron Beck and others, countless people have successfully learned to change their negative thoughts. This therapy approach is based upon the observation that how you feel is determined by what you think (Beck 1976). In other words, difficulties with depressed mood, irritability, and exaggerated anxiety are related to inaccurate and inflexible ways of interpreting life events. Cognitive therapy has been found to be effective in reducing heart rate and improving heart rate variability (Carney et al. 2000). It has also been rated highly in terms of overall satisfaction and goal attainment by heart patients (Edelman, Lemon, and Kidman 2003).

It is important to remember that you can change your negative thoughts without changing the real you. In fact, many people report that changing their negative thinking patterns brought them closer to their true selves.

The "ABC Thought Record" tool in this chapter is an effective way to begin to change your thinking. It will help you first observe your own thoughts and then shift toward more accurate thoughts. Various versions of this ABC format (also referred to as *daily thought records*) have been developed by cognitive therapists as a first step to help people learn how to make more accurate interpretations of events and reduce the assumptions or automatic thought habits that have been learned over time (Beck 1995; Newman 2003).

This thought-change tool can help you to correct your negative thoughts, just like putting on a new pair of glasses corrects your vision and helps you see more clearly. Try using this tool to increase your ability to think objectively, change your perspective, and see the positive results. As you practice the structured steps below, remember that changing negative thinking can have a large impact on many areas of your life—your mood, your relationships, and the things that you do for yourself. Scientific research has shown that cognitive therapy can be a powerful method for helping people to change negative thinking patterns and improve their emotional well-being (Hollon, DeRubeis, and Seligman 1992).

Changing negative thinking habits involves much more than just thinking positively. It means learning to look at and interpret a situation from a new and more accurate perspective. By using the steps below, you will learn to consider each situation from many different perspectives (including positive, negative, and neutral viewpoints) in order to reach more accurate and balanced conclusions.

ABC THOUGHT RECORD

Step 1: Record an emotionally distressing situation

Recall an event in which you experienced an emotional reaction. We will label this event A. Using the table below, write down a description of the event in column A. (You may want to copy this table in your journal in order to have more room to write, as well as for future use). Next, write down the thoughts that came into your mind in response to this event. We will label these thoughts B. Finally, write down the emotional reactions (C) that you had to this situation. (Ignore the fourth column for now.)

Situation or Event (A)	Thoughts Experienced (B)	Emotional Reactions (C)	Intensity Rating (1–10)

Look over the thoughts you recorded. Confronting your troubling thoughts may be uncomfortable, but try staying with this exercise. Review what you wrote down as the thoughts (B) associated with a specific situation (A) and the experience of negative emotions (C). Allow yourself to say the thoughts silently in your head and just observe them, notice them, become aware of them. These are thoughts that your mind has learned to say.

Step 2: Try to identify the thoughts as anxious, depressive, or angry

As you read over the thoughts that you wrote down, try to identify each as anxious, depressive, or angry. You may need to restate your thoughts more specifically. For example, one heart patient we know, Bill, after experiencing an argument with his wife, first wrote down, "I'm overwhelmed, stressed out." After we asked him to be a bit more specific, he wrote, "I'm afraid I'm going to lose it. I hate it when she acts so stupid. Nothing will ever change for the better." In the second group of thoughts, when Bill was more specific, he could actually identify fearful, hostile, and depressive thoughts.

Step 3: Rate the intensity of your emotional reaction

As you become aware of your emotions (C), rate them as mild, moderate, or intense. What was the intensity of the emotions you experienced in this situation? Rate your emotional intensity, with 1 indicating the mildest and 10 indicating the most distressing and intense. For example, Bill noted that he was angry (9), sad (8), and hopeless (10).

Step 4: Evaluate the accuracy of your thoughts

This step is also referred to as *guided self-discovery* and is adapted from the cognitive therapy approach developed by psychologists such as Judith Beck, Christine Padesky, and Dennis Greenberger. In this step, objectively consider the thoughts that you wrote down for their accuracy. Look for both supporting and disconfirming evidence. For example, in completing this step, Bill reviewed his thought *I hate it when she acts so stupid.* In reading this thought over carefully, he knew that his wife was not stupid or dull witted. In fact, she was an intelligent and competent professional. In realizing how inaccurate his thoughts were, Bill began to further understand what was really going on. More specifically, Bill realized that he gets frustrated when he has difficulty getting his wife to see his point of view. When they disagree, he feels vulnerable and scared. The thought that his wife is stupid serves to make him feel better about himself, but it does not help him communicate effectively. Instead, as Bill acts more aggressively toward her to compensate for these fears and feelings of vulnerability, his wife gets more fearful of his angry outbursts and finds it even more difficult to listen to Bill.

Returning to the thoughts (B) that you identified for yourself, now list any factual evidence that you think can support the accuracy of such thoughts. Getting evidence to support thoughts associated with strong negative emotions is not that easy. That's because many negative thoughts are based upon assumptions, not facts, and tend to be irrational, illogical, and inaccurate.

Next, write down the evidence that you can find that goes against your thoughts. Finding evidence that does not support your thoughts requires your willingness to see another viewpoint. Psychologists have developed questions that can help you identify ways in which the assumptions and statements you make to yourself are false. For example, Greenberger and Padesky (1995) suggest that you identify any experiences that show that the thought is not completely true all the time. In their book *Mind Over Mood*, they suggest thinking about what you would say to someone you care for who had the same thought, in order to better understand ways in which the thought is not 100 percent accurate. Other suggestions include asking family and friends for help by sharing the thought or assumption and asking them to provide disconfirming evidence. Others are more likely to be able to see a different side of the situation since they are not in it themselves.

Step 5: Develop more balanced thoughts about this situation

Balanced thoughts are those that describe facts about the situation more neutrally. For example, after objectively looking for both supporting and disconfirming evidence regarding his own thoughts, Bill developed more balanced thoughts: *I'm starting to get frustrated that she has difficulty seeing my viewpoint. But if I try, I can manage my reactions. I will try to communicate calmly to help change this situation for the better.*

Your previous thinking habits may have stopped you from thinking these more balanced thoughts in the past. However, you can develop new, balanced thoughts through the process of trying to find evidence for and against your negative thoughts.

Step 6: Repeat these balanced thoughts to yourself

These balanced thoughts will be more accurate, realistic, and optimistic descriptions of the situation. Remember that it took you many years to learn negative thinking habits. Therefore, it is likely to take practice and time to develop new patterns of thinking.

Step 7: Stop to notice how you are feeling after practicing your new thoughts in similar situations

Once again, note your thoughts and feelings about the situation and rate your negative feelings after changing your thoughts about the situation. For example, during Bill's next disagreement with his wife, he felt angry (with an intensity of 3), sad (5), and hopeless (2). The changes in ratings represent a significant improvement in his mood.

Step 8: Practice using your new balanced thoughts

Whenever you experience negative emotions or an increase in your distress level, use the ABC format to record your thoughts, to objectively evaluate your thoughts for accuracy by looking for supporting and disconfirming evidence, and to develop new, accurate, and balanced thoughts to practice under stressful situations. Such feelings of distress may be mild (for example, you find yourself mildly anxious while driving in traffic), moderate (for example, you notice that you are irritated and angry toward coworkers after a meeting), or very intense (for example, you find yourself extremely sad and hopeless following an argument with a family member).

REMEMBER THAT YOU CAN CHANGE YOUR NEGATIVE THINKING

Negative thinking habits are patterns of self-talk or internal dialogue that your mind has learned. Negative self-talk is usually automatic and is not very accurate. At best, it's based on a distortion of a few selected facts. When your perspective is distorted and narrow, it becomes very difficult to see the whole picture and understand both negative and positive aspects of a situation accurately. Such thinking is certainly not unique. Remember that many people engage in negative thinking. The important point here is to make a commitment to unlearning negative thought patterns and to practice thinking in more objective and accurate ways. You already experience your share of emotional pain when your thinking is accurate, because you, like everyone, experience stressful life situations. Why create additional distress—and stress on your heart—based upon distorted thoughts?

TRACK YOUR PROGRESS

By continuing to use the "ABC Thought Record," you can keep track of your progress by comparing your mood ratings from one situation to the next. If you experience any progress, don't forget to reward yourself! If you note a lack of positive change, you may be experiencing your current feelings as overwhelming. If so, using this tool in combination with other tools in this book—especially relaxation tools—can help you think more clearly. Remember that some improvement may result immediately, but big improvement comes with practice over time. Make a sincere commitment to try to change these thinking habits with all your heart.

13

Thinking Tool: Solving Stressful Problems

Simply being human means that you experience problems. In fact, you experience problems daily. Most of the time, these daily problems are small: losing your keys or not having exact change for the bus. Sometimes you experience daily problems that are more significant: difficulties with your boss or coworkers, not having enough money to pay the mortgage, or arguments with your spouse or friends. Even when problems appear small at the moment, they can create a lot of stress over time. You are better off if you are able to resolve them early on, before they begin to accumulate.

Life, unfortunately, presents you with bigger problems as well. These involve major events that radically change your overall quality of life: losing a job, getting a divorce, experiencing the death of a loved one, or becoming ill. Major events like these can create extreme stress in your life, particularly because they tend to create additional smaller problems. For example, experiencing heart disease can easily change a person's life. People who experience heart attacks or who receive a pacemaker or ICD consequently can experience emotional distress, a decrease in sexual drive, concerns about their future, a change in their overall activity level, relationship problems, financial difficulties, and so on. Both daily problems and major life events can cause stress.

PROBLEM SOLVING, STRESS, AND DISTRESS

We have spent collectively over forty years investigating the role that problem solving in daily life plays regarding both physical health and emotional health. Our research demonstrates that the more effective people are in resolving stressful problems that occur in everyday living, the more likely they are to be less depressed, be less anxious, be less angry, have fewer problems, and experience better health (Nezu 2004; Nezu, Wilkins, and Nezu 2004). In our research with patients experiencing varying types of heart problems, we have found a significant relationship between emotional distress and poor problem-solving skills (Nezu et al. 2004). In addition, Garcia and colleagues (1994) found that among men who suffered a heart attack, those who were most depressed and most anxious were also characterized by low usage of problem-solving strategies. Other mental-health professionals who work with cardiac patients have also strongly emphasized the need to teach heart patients problem-solving skills in order to improve their ability to cope with everyday stress and distress as a means of preventing further coronary problems (Burell 1996; Ewart 1990).

Therapists train people in problem-solving skills to help them with many different types of problems. For example, many scientific studies have shown that learning to solve daily problems can be an effective treatment for depression and anxiety. It is often part of effective treatments for interpersonal problems, anger, self-destructive behavior, and conduct problems in children. Finally, problem-solving training has been shown to significantly help people manage the problems and distress associated with having chronic medical or health problems like cancer, pain, obesity, difficulty stopping smoking, and substance abuse (D'Zurilla and Nezu 1999; Nezu et al. 2003; Nezu, Nezu, and Lombardo 2003).

EFFECTIVE PROBLEM SOLVING

Finding effective solutions to life's stressful problems usually involves a combination of two types of changes:

- overcoming barriers to adopting an optimistic attitude, and

- changing the problematic nature of an actual situation.

Adopting an Optimistic Attitude: The Role of Problem Orientation

Problem orientation refers to the manner in which you think about and feel about problems in general, as well as how successfully you cope with them. These thoughts and feelings can have a significant impact on your problem-solving efforts as well as on your emotional and physical well-being. Research has identified two problem-solving orientations: positive and negative (D'Zurilla, Nezu, and Maydeu-Olivares 2004).

Positive Problem Orientation

A positive orientation, which is associated with more successful problem solving, involves a general disposition to view a problem as a challenge rather than a threat, be optimistic and believe that problems are solvable, have the self-confidence to believe in your ability to be a successful problem solver, understand that solving difficult problems often takes persistence and effort, and commit yourself to solve the problem rather than avoid it.

Negative Problem Orientation

A negative orientation, which is associated with less successful problem solving, involves the general tendency to view a problem as being a major threat to your well-being, doubt your personal ability to solve a problem successfully, and generally become frustrated, upset, and emotionally distressed when confronted with problems.

Developing a positive problem orientation can enable you to successfully solve problems and cope with stressful situations. Substantial research has demonstrated that a negative orientation is associated with higher levels of depression, anxiety, anger, hopelessness, poor self-esteem, and pessimism (Nezu 2004). On the other hand, a strong positive orientation is associated with more successful problem resolution, more hopefulness, and better emotional health. Therefore, it is important to cultivate your ability to be optimistic.

We are not suggesting that you simply believe that life is a bowl of cherries. Rather, we suggest that you adopt the belief that problems are a normal part of life and that if you extend effort and give yourself time, you will be able to deal adequately with most of them. A better phrase is "realistic optimism"; that is, not blindly thinking that everything will be okay, but instead thinking that not everything will be all bad. Another way of looking at this is to think of the glass as half full rather than half empty, while also realizing that you want more liquid in the glass.

Overcoming Obstacles to Adopting a Positive Orientation

Certain obstacles may make it difficult for you to adopt a positive orientation. Such barriers include poor self-confidence, negative thinking, and negative emotional reactions.

If you believe that you tend to be an optimistic person in general, and you just want to learn some tips on effectively resolving stressful problems, you can skip ahead to the section in this chapter entitled "Changing the Nature of the Problem." However, if you think that your optimism needs a boost, continue reading this next section.

Overcoming Poor Self-Confidence: Visualizing Success

At times, lack of self-confidence can make you unable to see the light at the end of the tunnel. In other words, you may feel that you just can't see yourself successfully resolving a problem or achieving a particular goal. Through the technique of *visualization,* you can learn to become more optimistic by visualizing a positive outcome. Most people can learn to visualize. You visualize when you daydream, remember a past experience, picture an upcoming vacation in your mind, or think of people you know. Visualization is a powerful tool that can help you fulfill your dreams and achieve your life goals. It is very common for athletes to use visualization to improve their speed, strength, or performance. For example, gymnasts and skaters are taught to visualize a routine they will perform at a competition; basketball players are taught to visualize the ball going into the hoop. Practicing visualization actually improves their performance.

If lowered self-confidence is one of your potential barriers to successfully adopting a more optimistic attitude, you can use the "Visualizing Success" tool in chapter 18 as a means of overcoming this barrier.

Overcoming Negative Thinking: Learning the Rules of Healthy Thinking

We all think according to "rules" that are in our heads. The problem is that some of these rules are not very accurate, even though we have spent years learning them. Some of these rules operate without our day-to-day awareness. For example, what would you say if we asked you if you thought that it was realistic or possible for someone to be loved by everyone, 100 percent of the time? You would be correct in saying that of course this is not possible. Yet, every day, people allow themselves to feel badly and react with fear and surprise when they find out that someone does not like them. They become sad or angry over something that is unrealistic to expect in the first place. This can leave them feeling like they are constantly failing or not living up to their own expectations.

When you adopt the rules of healthy thinking, you can have a different outlook on life. Your happiness is much more in your control, because you focus on what you are doing, trying, achieving, and experiencing, not on what other people expect or how they react. The rules of healthy thinking are more accurate, objective, and rational. Many people have found these rules to be very helpful in decreasing feelings of anxiety and depression and in resolving problems with other people. These rules can help you manage stress and feel more confident and in control. They can also help you to adopt a more optimistic orientation toward solving problems.

How you think often affects the way you feel. How you feel about a situation is based on what you think about the situation. Situations don't make you anxious, depressed, or angry. It's what you say to yourself about the situation that leads you to feel a certain way. If you choose to interpret or think about situations differently, you will feel differently. For example, imagine that a coworker is not cooperating in finishing an assignment that you asked him to complete. You may interpret the situation to mean many different things: that the coworker has something against you, that he is lazy, that he believes your request to be foolish, that he didn't understand what you wanted him to do, that he had more respect for the previous person in your position than he has for you, that he is going through a very difficult personal crisis, or that he is afraid that his work won't be good enough so he's putting it off. Think about how each interpretation could result in very different emotions. The key is to focus on facts rather than assumptions. Remember that you can only change your own thoughts and behaviors. In this example, even if your coworker's behavior *is* based upon negative feelings toward you, this is a behavior that he, not you, must change.

Nothing's 100 percent perfect. You can't control the world, no matter how hard you try. The conditions for people or things to be perfect just don't exist. To say things should be otherwise is to believe in magic. They are what they are because of a long series of events, some of which include interpretations, responses from irrational self-talk, and so on. Sad or bad things happen, and life is not fairly balanced for all—that's just the way it is, as disappointing as that sounds. Accepting this fact will keep you focused on the goals that you set for yourself and keep you going despite periodic setbacks. Remember, if you don't try, nothing will ever get better. But life isn't problem free.

All humans make mistakes, even you. This is an inescapable fact. If you do not set reasonable goals for yourself and others, or allow for periodic "acts of stupidity," you greatly increase the chances of disappointment and unhappiness. However, if you do expect that you will make your fair share of mistakes and believe that these can actually become learning experiences, think of the opportunities you'll have for learning new skills. We all make mistakes! You can try hard not to make them, but you don't need to punish yourself when you do make a mistake.

Every minute you spend thinking negative thoughts takes away from the pleasure of focusing on positive aspects of your life. This rule highlights the fact that it is a personal choice to dwell on negative thoughts when there are often an equal number of positive thoughts available. Even if you are coping with a major loss such as the death of a loved one, positive thoughts and memories about the person or the relationship can be a focus of joy.

It takes two to have a bad relationship or conflict. Before launching into accusations and blame or thinking of yourself as an innocent victim, remember that with few exceptions, any person involved in an argument is contributing at least 30 percent to keeping it going. (If you read chapter 10, you'll recognize this as the 30 percent rule). Even if you have been unfairly accused or badly treated, there may be things that you could do differently to prevent this from happening in the future.

Forget winning—learning lasts longer. In contests where there is a winner, there is also a loser. Most people don't like to lose, so they get stuck on being the one who wins. The next time you face a difficult situation or conflict with someone, try to ask yourself, *Well, this is challenging. What can I learn from this situation?* Most often, you can learn something important, even if you don't win the argument or succeed in proving someone else wrong.

If, after wrestling with these rules, you continue to feel that your negative thinking blocks your ability to adopt an optimistic orientation, go to chapter 12 ("Changing Negative Thinking") for additional help.

Overcoming Negative Emotions

People experience upsetting feelings every day. However, emotions can be very tricky. Sometimes your feelings are a reaction to just one situation, and they simply pass. At other times, you are bothered by upsetting feelings for longer periods. Problems like depression, anxiety, anger, and bereavement all involve distressful feelings. If you find that such feelings currently make it difficult for you to adopt a positive orientation or if a strong emotional reaction hinders your ability to effectively resolve a particular problem, the following suggestions might help you to overcome this barrier.

Hold off making decisions while you're experiencing very intense emotions. Think of your emotions as a red light signaling that you are experiencing a problem that needs to be solved. This red light is telling you to stop and try to understand what is going on. It is very important that you don't immediately try to get rid of these negative feelings. Instead, take some time to understand these feelings before acting on them. Writing down your feelings or explaining them to someone who is objective can help you get a more balanced and accurate perspective on these problems.

Focus on one problem at a time. Some people are eager to solve all their problems at once. It is impossible to do this. In fact, good problem solvers will tell you that it is important to take on one problem at a time. With problems that are rather complex or especially stressful, it is usually a good idea to break them into smaller problems, ones that are a bit easier to tackle.

Reward yourself for the effort rather than the outcome. When you gain the ability to examine your strong emotions (such as fear, sadness, and anger) to help you understand the problems you are facing, be sure that you recognize the importance of taking this step and reward yourself for the effort. By using your feelings in this way and then following the problem-solving steps in the next section, you are likely to reduce the severity and number of problems in your life. Reward yourself as soon as you take the first step toward solving a problem, rather than expecting too much change all at once.

Try to focus on the future. Perhaps you dwell on past difficulties and hurts when you are feeling distressed, sad, anxious, or angry. These past difficulties can't be changed, and they can fuel negative feelings, turning your emotions into a bonfire. Instead, focus on what you would like to change in the future. Only use past problems, insults, and hurts to help you decide what goals or life changes are important now.

Practice relaxation and meditation. Chapters 14, 15, and 16 contain useful tools for quieting down your physical reactions so that you can think more clearly. Relaxation is more than getting away for the moment. True relaxation means creating a safe and peaceful mind. It is a time to be yourself and understand yourself better.

If you continue to have difficulties overcoming emotional barriers to adopting an optimistic orientation to problem solving, go to chapters 7 ("Using Feelings to Better Know Yourself") and 8 ("Expressing Emotions Constructively") for additional help.

CHANGING THE NATURE OF THE PROBLEM

Once you've adopted a more optimistic attitude toward problem solving, you're ready to move on to the next step: changing the problematic nature of a particular situation. Although many problems in life may appear complex and overwhelming, you can learn to solve your problems more effectively by using the guidelines outlined in this chapter. If you skipped over the section in this chapter on adopting an optimistic attitude, start with step 1 below. If you worked hard through that section to adopt a more positive orientation, then skip over step 1 and go straight to step 2.

SOLVING STRESSFUL PROBLEMS

The following six steps provide an overall method you can use to change the nature of a stressful situation so it is no longer a problem for you.

Step 1: Check your problem-solving attitude

Take a positive attitude toward solving your problem. The way you think about your problem can have a strong effect on what you actually do to solve it. In other words, if you believe that you should not avoid a problem and you are willing to try some creative thinking, then you can actually improve the situation. If you are having trouble developing or maintaining a positive problem-solving attitude or continue to believe that you can't learn to effectively solve problems, go back to the previous section.

Step 2: Understand the problem that you are trying to solve

There is actually scientific truth to the old saying that "a problem well defined is half solved." Problems that are vague or not clearly defined become more troublesome and frustrating than necessary. For instance, if you try to visit a friend in New York without further directions, you may wind up in Buffalo, Rochester, or Queens. Simply looking at a map without any specific destination or guidelines would be overwhelming, because there are many highways, roads, bridges, and tunnels that could lead you in many directions. You could end up in a dangerous or costly personal situation. However, if you define your destination by identifying a specific address, you will be able to set the best course for your travel. Here's how to define your problem and set realistic goals:

Get the facts. Try to get as much information about the problem as possible to better understand what is going on. Think of yourself as an investigative reporter or police detective.

Describe the facts in a clear language. For example, in describing a fearful situation, Jane said, "Riding in elevators is a nightmare. It's like I'm going to die or something!" A more accurate and factual description would be, "My anxiety is at its most intense when I ride in elevators. As the doors open and I step inside, my heart beats fast, my skin feels clammy, I get dizzy, and I have thoughts about dying. As soon as I step off, I feel relieved and my heart rate returns to normal." When you don't use clear language, you can blow things out of proportion or other people can misunderstand what you are saying. Reporters and detectives need to use clear language also.

Separate facts from assumptions. People make assumptions regularly without paying much attention to this automatic thought process. The difference between a fact and an assumption is that most people would independently agree that a fact is true. An assumption, on the other hand, is usually based upon a person's interpretation; two people would not necessarily agree. For example, let's say that two people both get a cold, bad-tasting cup of coffee in a restaurant. Both would agree that the coffee is cold. That is fact. However, one might assume that the cold coffee was a mistake and no harm was intended. The other person might make the assumption that the restaurant owner was trying to save money and served yesterday's coffee, not caring about the customers. Either one or both assumptions could be wrong. The only way to find out is to ask more questions and get the facts. Detectives, in solving mysteries, use facts rather than assumptions.

Identify what makes the situation a problem. Usually, a problem occurs when you are blocked in some way from getting what you want. This could be due to obstacles that are in the way, conflicting goals (ask anyone who wants to be a good parent and at the same time needs to earn an income for the family), reduced resources, recent changes, or actual losses.

Set realistic goals for changing the situation. This often means breaking down the problem into smaller parts, so that you can set reachable goals and approach different parts of the problem one at a time.

Now, in your journal or notebook, write down the problem you want to work on, remembering to

- gather all the facts

- use clear language

- separate facts from assumptions

- identify why the situation is a problem

- set realistic goals for changing the situation

After you describe your problem using these guidelines, you are ready to generate ideas about how to solve the problem.

Step 3: Brainstorm as many creative ideas as possible

Brainstorming involves listing as many alternatives or ideas to solve the problem as possible. It is important to write all of these ideas down. Even "silly" ideas should be written down, because they often lead to other ideas and good solutions. There are only three rules for learning to creatively brainstorm, but they are very important ones.

Quantity is important. Generate as many ideas as possible. If you feel like your ideas are starting to dry up, try combining or making small changes to previous ideas. Another way to add to your list is to imagine how a very creative person or a role model might think.

Don't judge. When you are making a list of ideas, hold off any criticism until you have completed your list. One sure way to stop your creative juices from flowing is to criticize yourself before you even have a chance to get all your ideas down.

Think of both general strategies and specific tactics. Strategies are general ways of solving a problem, while tactics are specific means of carrying them out. For example, if you were generating a list of ideas of how you could make up with a friend following an argument, one strategy might be to arrange a time to talk and tell him that you are sorry. Different tactics for carrying out the same strategy might include writing a letter, calling on the telephone, meeting for lunch, having another friend talk to him for you, and so forth. Put all of these down on your list.

Now, using these brainstorming rules, write down in your notebook a variety of possible solutions to the problem that you are working on.

Step 4: Make a decision about what solutions to use

Choose the ideas that are most likely to help you reach the goal that you set for yourself and the ideas that you are most likely to actually carry out. You can mark each idea with a rating of how likely it is to be effective (use a scale of 1 to 5, with 1 being very ineffective and 5 being very effective) and write some notes next to each alternative that you listed comparing the different consequences of each option. Weigh the positive and negative consequences and see which ideas come out better. It may be helpful to ask yourself the following questions when considering each alternative:

- Can I actually carry out this idea? If not, what do I need to do to be able to do this?

- Will this alternative meet my goals?

- Will this alternative be likely to overcome obstacles?

- What will be the consequences, both bad and good, of choosing this alternative?

- What will be the effect on me, my values, or my thoughts about myself if I choose this alternative?

- What will be the effect on people that I care about if I choose this idea?

- What will be the short-term consequences?

- What will be the long-term consequences?

As you ask yourself these questions, you will notice that some alternatives clearly have more advantages than others. Identify those ideas that have better consequences as possible ones to make up your solution plan.

Step 5: Develop a plan and carry out your decision

Choose those ideas that are rated 4 or 5. Develop a plan to carry out the solution. We all know that putting a plan into action can be hard to do. But you have done so much work up until now thinking about the best solution for you. Why stop now? It is important to write down your plan and give yourself a deadline for completing each step. Also, remember that the more arrows you shoot, the more likely you will hit the target. We first mentioned that idea to suggest that using many of the tools, rather than just one, will actually increase the likelihood that you will reach your ultimate goals. Here, the same idea applies: the more specific tactics that make up your solution plan, the more likely it is that you will solve any problem.

If you need help in motivating yourself to carry out the plan, here are some suggestions to get you started:

- Make a list of all the consequences of *not* solving the problem, as well as of successfully solving the problem. This will keep you mindful of all your good reasons for putting a plan into action.

- Picture yourself carrying out the plan successfully. You may find it helpful to use the "Visualizing Success" tool we'll teach you in chapter 18.

- Post a daily reminder with a slogan or personal motivation statement in a spot that you frequently see (for example, your refrigerator). We know one person who borrowed the "Just do it!" slogan from a famous sporting goods company, stuck it on his refrigerator, and found it helpful as a reminder every time he passed by it.

Step 6: Monitor your progress

Compare what you thought would happen with what actually happened. If the outcome was satisfactory, you know that you have successfully applied your problem-solving skills. If it was not, try again with a different plan, going through all the steps.

You might feel that these six steps are a lot of work to do when solving your daily problems. However, remember that the more you practice, the easier it becomes to use this technique and the faster the results. In general, you should use all the steps when dealing with complex or difficult problems. By doing so, you will make these problems less stressful.

REWARD YOURSELF

Solving problems is sometimes hard work. You should reward yourself for your effort. Remember that it is especially important to reward yourself for trying, not for finding the perfect solution or not having problems. As human beings, we will always have day-to-day problems as well as major problems. Think about the long-term benefits if you solve your day-to-day problems just 25 percent more effectively. Most people using the problem-solving tool report much more benefit than this.

Problem-solving skills represent a tool that you can use to resolve problems and difficulties encountered in daily living. In a way, by learning how to solve day-to-day problems, you can learn to be your own counselor or therapist. In addition, by using the steps you learned in this chapter, you can get started on reducing your distress and improving the quality of your life. Learning to solve daily problems can be an effective treatment for depression, anxiety, and anger. When you face problems, you experience a whole range of feelings, and it is important to learn how to stop these feelings from consuming you.

14

Relaxation Tool: Deep Breathing

If you are like most people, you take breathing for granted, and you may not realize the "medicine" that you carry within yourself all of the time, every day. With each breath of air you take in, you give your body the oxygen it needs, and with each breath you release, you get rid of carbon dioxide. Remember that the heart and the lungs depend on each other. The right side of your heart pumps blood into your lungs. It is in the lungs that the blood receives oxygen and gets rid of carbon dioxide. The newly oxygenated blood goes from the lungs to the left part of your heart, which pumps it to the rest of your body, delivering oxygen to the cells. Blood that returns from the tissues of your body to the right heart chambers needs to circulate through your lungs before it enters the left side of your heart.

Although breathing seems to be a simple and automatic activity, how you breathe can have extremely important consequences for your heart health. Did you know that there are different types of breathing? For example, there are spiritual rituals that involve breathing meditations that help people maintain a sense of awareness and appreciate the flow of life that is always present, whether or not we are conscious of it.

DO YOU SUFFER FROM "BAD BREATH"?

By "bad breath" we mean the type of breathing that works *against* your heart health rather than *for* your heart health. Certain types of breathing can be especially good for you. Psychologists have shown that when you learn how to breathe slowly and regularly, you can quiet your mind by helping your body to relax. Further, there is scientific evidence that deep and rhythmic breathing can also improve the rhythms of your heart. This change in heart rate rhythm can lead to a reduced risk of cardiac events. Research suggests that the use of a combination of focused breathing and positive mental states is an effective method of offsetting negative mental and physical reactions to daily stressors (McCraty et al. 1995).

DEEP BREATHING

Breathing for your health and well-being requires you to breathe from your abdominal or "stomach" area. This type of breathing is also referred to as *diaphragmatic breathing* and is very different than breathing from your chest area. *Chest breathing* often occurs when you experience even mild stress. It is irregular, rapid, and shallow breathing. In some cases, when people are very scared or upset, they may actually hold their breath. Other people breathe so fast that they hyperventilate and can actually pass out. This is what we mean by "bad breath." Breathing improperly can contribute to many problems, such as high blood pressure, panic attacks, muscle tension, tiredness, headaches, and negative moods.

Abdominal or deep diaphragmatic breathing, on the other hand, is the type of natural breathing babies do; it is also how relaxed, resting adults breathe. Singers use abdominal breathing to get the most out of their voices. Abdominal breathing can also be used for pain management; the panting form of breathing used by women during childbirth is one example. Diaphragmatic breathing is one of the simplest, cheapest, and safest ways to help your body calm down. Breathing is an incredibly powerful health tool that you have available to you at all times.

It is not surprising, therefore, that deep, diaphragmatic breathing can be helpful in cardiac rehabilitation and in treating a wide range of heart problems, including essential hypertension and angina (Gilbert 2003). Often in combination with other tools like the ones we teach in this book, deep breathing has been used to reduce anxiety, panic, depression, irritability, anger problems, muscle tension, headaches, and fatigue.

Get Ready to Monitor Your Progress

When you are applying this deep breathing technique, it is important to monitor your progress. *SUDS* stands for *subjective units of distress*, a numbering system to describe the level of tension, pain, or distress that a person experiences. Using a ten-point scale, where 1 represents the lowest level of distress and 10 represents the highest, try rating yourself right now.

Monitoring your SUDS level just means taking a moment to rate your level of distress before and after each time you engage in a breathing exercise. Over time, you will see the benefits of your deep breathing reflected in lower SUDS ratings. Now you are ready to learn how to breathe in ways that are helpful to your heart health—as if your life depended upon it.

DEEP BREATHING

To practice diaphragmatic breathing, locate a quiet and comfortable place in your home for the initial practice sessions. After a while, you can practice anywhere. While breathing exercises can begin to show benefits in a few minutes, the best way to achieve the most profound and long-lasting effects is to practice two to three minutes, once or twice each day.

Step 1: Record your SUDS level

Take out your journal or notebook and write down your SUDS level before beginning the deep breathing exercise. Be sure to note the date so you can monitor your progress over time.

Step 2: Position yourself comfortably

Now lie down or sit in a comfortable position and close your eyes. Put your right hand on your belly, just under your rib cage and about even with your waistline. Put your left hand on the center of your chest, just under your neck.

Step 3: Become aware of your breathing

Notice how you are breathing. Which hand rises the most? If the hand on your belly is moving up and down, then you are breathing more from your diaphragm or abdomen. This is the best way to breathe. Practice doing this now, keeping your hand on your belly. As you take in your breath, imagine that your entire abdomen is a balloon filling up with air. When you exhale, let all the air out of your belly slowly and feel it collapse just like a balloon that is letting out air.

Step 4: Breathe deeply for five minutes

Inhale slowly and deeply through your nose into your abdomen, filling all the spaces in your belly with air. (If you have difficulty breathing through your nose, go ahead and breathe through your mouth.)

Now exhale through your mouth, making a quiet whooshing sound like the wind as you gently and slowly blow out. Purse your lips, forming an O, and release your breath, as if you were trying to make a paper sailboat glide slowly across the water. Take long, slow, deep breaths.

Feel your belly rise and fall.

Repeat a phrase (silently or out loud) with each breath, such as "I take in life" with each breath in and "I am giving life" with each breath out. You could also say "I am taking in a good breath" and "Now I am releasing the tension." Can you think of others?

Continue to breathe this way for approximately five minutes.

Step 5: Record your SUDS rating

At the end of each breathing session, scan your body for tension or negative feelings such as anxiety or anger, and record your SUDS level.

THE WELLNESS BREATH

Although the deep breathing exercise takes only five minutes and therefore fits into most schedules, you may want to try an additional breathing exercise, *the wellness breath*, which can be practiced anywhere, anytime.

Andrew Weil, a physician well-known for promoting the idea that people can tap into their own strengths in order to better manage their health, once told a group of people gathered at one of his lectures that he was going to reveal the "secret" of one of the most powerful medicines available (Weil 1996). Intrigued by this announcement, everyone paid close attention. Dr. Weil stood up, took a big breath from his diaphragm, and exhaled fully. Although his demonstration was fun, he had a very serious message: the power of even one deep breath should not be underestimated.

THE WELLNESS BREATH

Follow these steps to refresh your body, keep your breathing apparatus in good shape, and actually increase mental alertness.

Step 1: Begin by standing up straight (watch your posture).

Step 2: Slowly inhale a complete and full natural breath from the pit of your abdomen. Hold this for a few seconds.

Step 3: Pretend that you are blowing through a straw and exhale slowly but with force through the small opening in your lips. Stop exhaling for a second and then blow out a bit more air. Continue this process until you have blown out all the air in brief, forceful puffs.

Step 4: Resume normal breathing.

FINAL THOUGHTS

Deep breathing is a simple and effective way to calm down your body and feel relaxed. We recommend that you use the breathing tools in combination with the other anxiety reduction or stress management tools in this book. When you try the techniques in this chapter, remember to breathe from your abdomen or belly, not your chest. Remember to take deep, slow breaths, not quick, shallow ones. You can't do two opposite things at the same time: you can't breathe rapidly while breathing slowly. In other words, you can't be anxious or angry while simultaneously feeling relaxed.

15

Relaxation Tool: Autogenic Training

Autogenic training was developed over fifty years ago by the German physician Johannes Schultz as a technique to calm the mind and body and help people learn to let go of physical and psychological tension. Being able to achieve this type of relaxed body state is an extremely important skill for learning to create balance in your body's energies and to help you face the challenge of changing your thoughts, feelings, and actions in the direction of heart health. In its most basic form, autogenic training is a relaxation method based on passive concentration on bodily perceptions that are facilitated by self-suggestions. This relaxation approach has been found to be very effective in both calming the mind and body and improving a variety of medical conditions, including coronary heart disease (Stetter and Kupper 2002).

TRAINING YOURSELF IN SELF-HYPNOSIS

Autogenic training is a powerful form of self-hypnosis that includes focusing your mental attention on feelings of heaviness, fostering a sense of warmth in your arms and legs, and focusing attention on your breathing. Your attitude toward the exercises should not be intense or strenuous but more like *I'm going to tell my body to do this and just let it happen.* This tool uses simple phrases that help the body relax and encourage specific physical reactions to occur. For example, the phrase "My arms are heavy and warm" can increase blood flow to the hands and feet and indirectly slow down your heart rate.

This relaxation tool is considered to be a combination of meditation and self-hypnosis. Remember that this is not the popular kind of "hypnosis" that encourages people to act differently (like a chicken, for example). Rather, you control what you are doing at all times, remain fully conscious but relaxed, and have the experience of heightened attention. You will be able to tune out external stimuli or events and focus on the topic at hand. When in this physical state, you are able to prompt changes in your own body that can release tension, create a calm state of mind, and ultimately care for your heart by reducing negative arousal related to your anxiety and anger.

AUTOGENIC TRAINING IS EFFECTIVE

Autogenic training has many applications to improve mental and physical health. It is a powerful relaxation strategy that is used to help calm and manage negative emotions such as anger, anxiety, and depression; to foster relaxation; and to stimulate creativity and positive emotions. Autogenic training can help alleviate emotional pain and help you to accomplish your goals of relaxation; it has also been found to be effective in relieving a variety of physical symptoms. These include migraine headaches and other chronic pain problems, infertility, insomnia, asthma, eczema, premenstrual syndrome, gastrointestinal disorders, Raynaud's disease, and coronary heart disease (Stetter and Kupper 2002). With regard to coronary heart disease, research has demonstrated that autogenic training can successfully lower blood pressure in patients diagnosed with hypertension (Rossi et al. 1989), improve cardiovascular reactivity (Haugen 2000), and decrease depression and anxiety in patients who experienced a myocardial infarction (Polackova, Bockova, and Sedivec 1982). Taken together, research evidence from studies around the world indicates that autogenic training can be a particularly useful strategy in improving both physical symptoms and the negative psychological symptoms that can harm your heart.

AUTOGENIC TRAINING

You can have a friend or family member with a calming voice make a recording of the script provided in the following paragraphs, or you may want to make the recording yourself. Be sure to read softly and slowly, pausing where indicated in the script. You can even add some of your favorite relaxing instrumental music playing softly in the background. This way, you will have your own autogenic training recording that you can use over and over again.

Find a comfortable location to practice, such as a recliner, couch, bed, or soft floor covering. Remember to loosen your clothing, remove glasses or contact lenses, and lower the lights to create a more calming environment. Make sure that your legs are not crossed and your head is supported, as your body is likely to experience a sense of heaviness that would be uncomfortable if your legs or arms were in a crossed position. A single session will take about twenty to twenty-five minutes to complete.

Practice once every day for at least one week. Practicing this tool is important. As with learning any other skill (for example, driving a car, using a computer, or playing piano), the more you practice, the better you get. Trying this exercise only once or twice will not produce the kind of results that lead to significant reductions in anxiety or negative arousal.

Prior to beginning the exercise, assess your body for any signs of muscle tension. If you discover that a site is particularly tense, concentrate on it during the exercise. In this manner, you can become aware of the specific ways in which this training is helping you to calm your mind and body.

Now get comfortable and follow the script below.

Autogenic Training Script

Let yourself go now, getting deeply relaxed all over. Start by taking a deep breath, feeling the air flow in, way down to your lower belly, and filling your whole abdominal region. Now exhale slowly, and as you do, feel the air slowly releasing from your abdomen and allow yourself to float down into the surface you are sitting or lying on. Close your eyes and focus on the sensations of breathing. Imagine your breath rolling in and out like waves coming onto the shore. Think quietly to yourself, My breath is calm and effortless, calm and peaceful. Repeat this phrase to yourself as you imagine waves of relaxation flowing through your body . . . through your chest and shoulders, into your arms and back, into your hips and legs. Feel a sense of tranquillity moving through your entire body. Continue this for the next few moments. (Reader: pause for ten seconds.)

This is your time. Do not waste it on thoughts of what you should be doing later or what you did earlier. Focus only on your own internal voice and what your body is feeling right now. If you find that thoughts intrude, do not dwell on them. You can simply notice them, let them pass, and come back to your own inside voice. Let them pass like clouds in the sky. Imagine a white light starting at the crown of your head. The light is your inner energy, your mind's eye, and it will travel and spread warmth wherever you tell it to.

Right now, travel with your mind's eye down to your right shoulder into your right arm and into your right hand. Make mental contact with it. Feel it, be aware of it, and notice where it makes contact with the surface it's resting on. Allow your hand to become heavy and very warm. Imagine warmth flowing gently through your hand, wrist, and fingers. (Reader: pause for ten seconds.)

Maintain this contact and repeat silently to yourself, My right hand is heavy. My right hand is heavy and warm. My right hand is letting go. Repeat these phrases to yourself for the next several seconds. As you maintain contact with that hand, allow your whole right arm to now become heavy and warm. Continue to breathe regularly and slowly, saying these three phrases silently to yourself now: My right arm is heavy. My right arm is heavy and warm. My right arm is

letting go. For the next thirty seconds, say them over and over in your head.
(Reader: pause for thirty seconds.)

Note what your arm feels like now. Is it tingling or heavy? Does it feel hollow? Is it light and floating? What does it feel like? Become aware of any tiny sensations and try to describe them to yourself. Now, using the image of the white light, your mind's eye, focus on your right arm again. Make mental contact with it. Just allow it to do the things that you say. Repeat again to yourself, My right arm is heavy. My right arm is heavy and warm. My right arm is letting go. For the next several seconds, ignore all other thoughts and repeat these three phrases over and over again. (Reader: pause for thirty seconds.)

What does your right arm feel like? Carefully scan it with your mind's eye. Try to describe, silently to yourself, exactly what it feels like. Think to yourself, If I had to describe what my arm feels like right now, what would I say? Is there any sensation at all?

As you allow your right arm to stay completely relaxed, travel with your mind's eye up your right arm, across your shoulders, and down to your left arm and hand. Make mental contact with it; notice where it rests on the surface below. Allow it to become very heavy and warm. Imagine warmth spreading and flowing gently through your arm, wrist, hand, and fingers. Maintain this contact and repeat silently to yourself, My left arm is heavy. My left arm is heavy and warm. My left arm is letting go. Repeat these phrases silently for the next few moments. (Reader: pause for thirty seconds.)

As you maintain contact with that arm and continue breathing regularly and slowly, say these three phrases silently to yourself now: My left arm is heavy. My left arm is heavy and warm. My left arm is letting go. For the next thirty seconds, say them over and over to yourself. (Reader: pause for thirty seconds.)

Note what your arm feels like right now. Is it tingling? Does it feel heavy and warm? Is it light or floating? What does it feel like? Become aware of any tiny sensations and try to describe them to yourself. (Reader: pause for ten seconds.)

Think to yourself, If I had to describe to someone else exactly what my arm and hand feel like, how would I describe it? Silently use the words to describe it to yourself for a few seconds. (Reader: pause for ten seconds.)

Once again, focus your attention on your left arm. Make mental contact with it. Just allow it to do the things that you say. Say again to yourself over and over, My left arm is heavy. My left arm is heavy and warm. My left arm is letting go. For the next thirty seconds, ignore all other thoughts and repeat these three phrases over and over again. (Reader: pause for thirty seconds.)

What does your right arm feel like? Carefully scan both arms with your mind's eye. Do you notice any differences between the right and the left? Is there any spot of tension in either arm? If so, just allow the light of your mind's eye to spread total warmth and relaxation throughout both arms and hands. Try to verbalize to yourself exactly what it feels like. Is there any sensation at all? (Reader: pause for thirty seconds.)

Now bring your mental focus to your legs for a few moments. Imagine your mind's eye spreading a light of warmth and heaviness that flows from your arms down into your legs. Think to yourself, My legs are becoming heavy. Warmth is flowing through my feet, down into my toes. My legs and feet are heavy and warm. My legs and feet are letting go. (Reader: pause for ten seconds.)

Now scan your body for any points of tension, and if you find some, let those areas go limp and allow your muscles to become completely relaxed. Notice how heavy, warm, and limp your body has become. Think to yourself, All of my muscles are letting go. I'm getting more and more relaxed. (Reader: pause for fifteen seconds.)

Take a deep breath. Feel the air as it gently fills your lungs down to your belly. As you breathe out, say to yourself, I am calm. I am at peace. I am warm and relaxed. Use whatever words help you to become relaxed. Do this for a few moments and feel the sense of warmth and calm throughout your body. (Reader: pause for ten seconds.)

Now imagine counting to three, and with each number, take a slow, deep breath, then exhale. On the count of three, slowly open your eyes and allow yourself to get accustomed to the room. Stretch your arms and legs before rising and returning to your activities. (Reader: pause ten seconds.) *One ... slowly get more used to your surroundings and know where you are. Two ... bring back with you all the feelings of relaxation and calmness, even though you are becoming more alert ... and three.*

TRACK YOUR PROGRESS

As you learn and practice autogenic training, assess your tension level before and after each practice session. You can use the SUDS method described in the previous chapter to monitor your progress. You may want to keep notes regarding each session, especially when you are first learning how to use this technique. There may be times when you have a bit of difficulty sustaining your attention, or your mind may wander off. These experiences are normal and will lessen with time as you continue to practice. Don't be discouraged if you don't feel calm or relaxed after one or two attempts. The more you practice, the more successful you will be in helping yourself maintain a calm body and mind. The benefits of using relaxation tools such as autogenic training are similar to those of physical exercise or taking vitamins. The biggest payoff to your mind and heart will be evident after continued use and practice, because you will have developed a habit and conditioned your body to create a calm physical state.

16

Relaxation Tool: Deep Muscle Relaxation

Deep muscle relaxation, also known as *progressive muscle relaxation*, was first described in the early twentieth century by Edmund Jacobsen, a Chicago physician, as a technique to reduce physiological tension in the muscles. Since that time, many physicians and psychologists have come to believe that this is a very important tool to enhance both physical and mental health. The current theory behind how it works is based on the idea that when you experience anxious thoughts or feelings, your body responds with muscle tension. This tension in the muscles then gets interpreted by your brain as a signal of more anxiety. Thus begins a vicious cycle between mind and body.

Progressive relaxation releases muscle tension and gives a feeling of warmth and well-being to the body. Your brain interprets this relaxation to mean that everything is okay. It is impossible to have your body physically relaxed and feel anxious or tense at the same time. Deep muscle relaxation, when successfully learned, can be a very strong natural antistress medicine and break the vicious cycle.

MUSCLE RELAXATION TRAINING IS EFFECTIVE

Muscle relaxation training has been evaluated in many research studies and found to be an important tool for overall stress management (Ferguson 2003). Excellent results have been found for the treatment of muscle tension and spasms, insomnia, depression, fatigue, irritable bowel syndrome, chronic pain, high blood pressure, and many different types of anxiety problems, including fears and phobias. In other words, it is a very powerful tool. With regard to cardiovascular disease, Haaga and colleagues (1994) found progressive muscle relaxation to be effective in reducing psychophysiological reactivity and outward anger expression in men with borderline hypertension. Further studies found similar results for women with hypertension (Hahn et al. 1994) and adults undergoing cardiac rehabilitation (Cole, Pomerleau, and Harris 1993)—that is, relaxation training led to significant decreases in both systolic and diastolic blood pressure for both sets of patients. Loewe and colleagues (2002) more recently found progressive muscle relaxation training to be effective regarding both emotional and physical well-being among a group of patients who recently experienced a heart attack. Collectively, these results suggest strongly that deep muscle relaxation is an effective strategy to reduce negative emotions and therefore improve heart health.

LEARNING DEEP MUSCLE RELAXATION

Essentially, progressive muscle relaxation will teach you to initially tense a particular muscle group (for example, your left hand) and then to release that tension in order to feel relaxed and calm. You will progress in a similar manner throughout all muscle groups in your entire body. You will then learn to foster a sense of overall relaxation without tensing any muscles.

Read through the relaxation induction script to better understand what we mean when we tell you to tense a particular muscle. Note that you should not tense your muscles in such a way as to cause cramping or pain. Rather, tense the muscle in order to feel the tension. Also, try to concentrate on the particular muscle group that is being addressed and not any others. For example, when asked to make a fist, do so simply by clenching your hand into a fist, not by raising your entire arm. Try practicing these tense-relax exercises before you actually engage in the relaxation induction for the first time so that you can get the maximum effect possible.

You'll want to make a recording of the progressive muscle relaxation script. You can make the recording yourself, or you can ask a friend or family member whose voice is soothing to you. Remember to read softly and slowly and pause where indicated in the script. Consider including relaxing music in the background.

Choose a comfortable place to practice this relaxation technique: a recliner, couch, bed, or carpeted floor. Loosen your clothing, remove glasses or contact lenses, and dim the lights. Make sure that your legs are not crossed and your head is supported. As your body relaxes, you will experience a sense of heaviness that would be uncomfortable if your legs or arms were crossed. Practice once every day for at least one week. A single session will take about twenty-five to thirty minutes to complete.

Progressive muscle relaxation is a skill, and as with any other skill, the more you practice, the better you get. Trying this strategy only once or twice will not produce the kind of results that lead to significant reductions in anxiety or negative arousal.

PROGRESSIVE MUSCLE RELAXATION

Before each session, notice any areas of your body that are particularly tense. You'll want to pay special attention to these parts as you go through the exercise. This will help you become aware of the specific ways in which this training is helping you to calm your mind and body.

Progressive Muscle Relaxation Script

Let yourself go now, getting deeply relaxed all over. Start by taking a deep breath, feeling the air flow in, way down to your lower belly, and filling your whole abdominal region. Now exhale slowly, and as you do, feel the air slowly releasing from your lower abdomen and allow yourself to float down into the surface you are sitting or lying on. Close your eyes and focus on the sensations of breathing. Imagine your breath rolling in and out like waves coming onto the shore.

Think quietly to yourself, I am going to let go of tension. I will relax and smooth out my muscles. I will feel all of the tightness and the tension dissolve away.

Now we will begin the progressive muscle relaxation procedure. Your first muscle group will be your hands, forearms, and biceps.

First, clench your right fist, tighter and tighter. Study the tension and discomfort as you do so. Keep it clenched and notice the tension in your fist, hand, and forearm. Hold this tension in your right fist for a few seconds. (Reader: pause for three seconds.) *Now relax. Feel the looseness in your right hand. Notice the contrast with the tension. Repeat the procedure with your right fist, noticing as you relax that this is the opposite of tension. Relax and feel the difference.*

Now clench your left fist, tighter and tighter. Study the tension and discomfort as you do so. Keep it clenched and notice the tension in your fist, hand, and forearm. Hold this tension in your left fist for a few seconds. (Reader: pause for three seconds.) *Now relax. Feel the looseness in your left hand. Notice the contrast with the tension.* (Reader: pause for five seconds.)

Now repeat the entire procedure with your left fist (Reader: pause for five seconds), *then both fists at once. Clench both fists, tighter and tighter, studying the tension and discomfort as you do so. Keep them clenched and notice the tension. Hold this tension in both fists now for a few seconds.* (Reader: pause for three seconds.) *Now relax. Feel the looseness in your hands. Allow warmth and relaxation to spread all over.*

Now bend your elbows in order to tense your biceps. Tense them now and observe the feeling of tension and tightness. (Reader: pause for three seconds.) *Now relax. Let your arms straighten out. Let relaxation flow in, and feel the difference between the tension and strain in your arms when they were tensed and how they felt when they were relaxed, loose, and limp. Now repeat this procedure. Bend your elbows and tense your biceps. Tense them now and observe the feeling of discomfort.* (Reader: pause for three seconds.) *Now relax. Let your arms straighten out. Let* relaxation flow in, and feel the difference between the tension and strain in your arms when they were tensed and how they felt when they were relaxed.

Your next muscle group will be your head, face, and scalp. Turning attention to your head, wrinkle your forehead. (Reader: pause for three seconds.) Now relax and smooth it out. Imagine that your entire scalp is becoming smooth and relaxed . . . at peace . . . at rest. Now frown and notice the tightness and strain spreading throughout your forehead. (Reader: pause for three seconds.) Now let go. Allow your brow to become smooth and soft again. Close your eyes now and squeeze them tighter. Notice the tension, the discomfort. (Reader: pause for three seconds.) Now relax your eyes and allow them to remain gently closed. (Reader: pause for three seconds.) Now clench your jaw. Bite down like you're trying to hold something in your teeth. (Reader: pause for three seconds.) Now relax your jaw. When your jaw is relaxed, your lips may be slightly parted and you may feel your tongue loosely in your mouth. Now press your tongue against the roof of your mouth. Feel the ache it creates in the back of your mouth. (Reader: pause for three seconds.) Now relax. Feel your tongue soft and loose in your mouth. Now purse your lips into an O as if you were blowing bubbles. (Reader: pause for three seconds.) Now relax your lips. Notice that your forehead, scalp, eyes, jaw, tongue, and lips are all relaxed. (Reader: pause for five seconds.)

Your next muscle group will be your head, neck, and shoulders. Press your head back as far as you can and observe the tension in your neck. Roll it from right to left and notice the changing location of the stress. Now bend your head forward, pressing your chin to your chest. Feel the tension in your throat and the back of your neck. (Reader: pause for three seconds.) Now relax. Allow your head to return to a comfortable position. Let the relaxation spread over your shoulders. (Reader: pause for three seconds.) Now shrug your shoulders. Keep the tightness and tension as you hunch your head down between your shoulders. Feel how uncomfortable this position is. (Reader: pause for three seconds.) Now relax your shoulders. Drop them back and feel relaxation spreading throughout your neck, throat, and shoulders—pure relaxation, deeper and deeper. (Reader: pause for five seconds.)

Your next muscle group will be your chest and abdomen. First, give your entire body a chance to relax. Feel the comfort and the heaviness. Now breathe in and fill your lungs completely. Hold your breath and notice the tension. (Reader: pause for three seconds.) Now exhale. Let your chest and abdomen become loose while the air is coming out. Continue relaxing and let your breathing become calm and natural. (Reader: pause for three seconds.) Repeat the deep breath once more and notice the tension leave your body as you exhale. (Reader: pause for five seconds.)

Now tighten your stomach as if you are trying to suck it in and make it hard and flat. Hold it. (Reader: pause for three seconds.) Notice the tension. Now relax. Arch your back without straining. Notice the tension in your lower back and hold this position for a few seconds. (Reader: pause for three seconds.) Focus on the tension in your lower back. Now relax, gently lowering your back down and relaxing all over. (Reader: pause for five seconds.)

Your next muscle group will be your legs and buttocks. Tighten your buttocks and thighs. Flex your thighs by pressing down on your heels. (Reader: pause for three seconds.) *Now relax and feel the difference.* (Reader: pause for three seconds.) *Now point your toes like a ballet dancer and make your calves tense. Study the tension and hold it.* (Reader: pause for three seconds.) *Now relax. Notice the difference between the relaxed feeling in your legs and the discomfort that you experienced a moment ago. Bend your toes toward your face, creating tension in your shins. Pause and hold it.* (Reader: pause for three seconds.) *Now relax again.* (Reader: pause for five seconds.)

Feel the heaviness and warmth throughout your lower body as the relaxation spreads all over you. Relax your feet, ankles, calves, shins, knees, thighs, and buttocks. Now let the relaxation spread to your stomach, lower back, and chest. (Reader: pause for three seconds.) *Let go more and more.* (Reader: pause for three seconds.) *Experience the relaxation deepening in your shoulders, arms, and hands. Deeper and deeper. Notice the feeling of looseness and relaxation in your neck, jaw, and all your facial muscles.* (Reader: pause for three seconds.) *Say to yourself, My muscles are relaxed, warm, and smooth. I am letting go of all my tension. I am deeply relaxed. My muscles are relaxed, warm, and smooth. I am letting go of all my tension. I am deeply relaxed. Enjoy these feelings of relaxation for the next few moments.* (Reader: pause for two minutes, during which you can occasionally say, "More and more relaxed, deeper and deeper into a state of relaxation.")

Now bring your focus back to the present time and place while I count from one to five. With each increasing number, try to become more alert to your surroundings. Open your eyes, but keep the feelings of relaxation in your body. (Reader: slowly count from one to five.)

TRACK YOUR PROGRESS

To keep track of your progress, assess your tension level before and after each practice session. You can use the SUDS method described in chapter 14 to monitor your progress. You may want to use your journal to keep notes regarding each session, especially as you are first learning progressive muscle relaxation. Don't worry if you have trouble staying focused or your mind wanders. This will happen less often as you continue to practice. Don't become discouraged if this exercise doesn't seem to work the first time or two. The more you practice, the more successful you will be in generating a calm mental and physical state. As with physical exercise, the benefits of using relaxation tools will become apparent over time. Essentially, you are conditioning your body to create a calm state.

17

Visualization Tool: Mind Travel to a Safe Place

Everybody visualizes or uses their imagination. Daydreaming, remembering, anticipating a future event, or thinking of someone you know requires you to visualize. Visualization can be a powerful tool for changing your life. Five minutes of visualization can cancel out hours, days, or even weeks of negative thinking. Several sessions a day can change a habit that took years to form and become entrenched. This tool helps you to improve your existing powers of visualization so that you can practice and use them to increase a sense of peace and wellness in your life. We will provide a set of instructions that guide your visualization as a means of reducing anxiety and negative arousal. That is why another term for this approach is *guided imagery*.

Visualization is the conscious and intentional creation of mental impressions that use all your five senses (seeing, hearing, smelling, touching, and tasting) for the purpose of changing your feelings, thoughts, and behavior. People use visualization for different reasons. The purpose of the visualization tool we'll teach in this chapter is to create a safe place in your mind. You can go there to relax, feel safe and secure, let go, and completely be yourself. In times of stress, this technique can be extremely helpful in reducing distress. This tool can also put you in a relaxed state of mind in anticipation of a stressful event (for example, asking your boss for a raise).

VISUALIZATION IS EFFECTIVE

Visualization can be a very effective tool for many stress-related physical and psychological problems, including depression, headaches, muscle spasms, chronic pain, and anxiety problems (Nezu, Nezu, and Lombardo 2004). It is known to be a potent intervention to improve the quality of life of cancer patients (Spiegel and Moore 1997) and in reducing pain (Eller 1999). Pleasant guided imagery has also been found to relieve negative moods and improve depression (Skeie, Skeie, and Stiles 1989). A recent study where guided imagery was compared to medication to reduce pain associated with fibromyalgia demonstrated that visualization was significantly more effective than either amitriptyline or placebo (Fors, Sexton, and Götestam 2002). Visualization has also been successful in helping patients faced with cardiovascular problems cope more effectively (Achterberg et al. 2003).

LEARNING VISUALIZATION

You can have a friend or family member with a soothing voice make a recording of the script below, or you may want to make the recording yourself. Remember to read softly and slowly. You can even add relaxing instrumental music in the background. Once you've recorded the script, you will have your own guided imagery recording that you can use over and over again.

You can practice visualization in a recliner or on a couch, bed, or carpeted floor. Remember to loosen your clothing, remove glasses or contact lenses, and lower the lights to create a calm environment. Practice once every day for at least one week. A single session will take fifteen to twenty minutes.

Like the relaxation exercises you learned in previous chapters, visualization is a skill. You will get better at it the more you do it. Trying this technique only once or twice won't yield the same results as long-term practice.

VISUALIZATION SCRIPT

Use short, positive statements or affirmations when you begin your visualization. Examples include

- *I can relax.*

- *I will let the tension and anxiety go.*

- *I have peace within myself.*

Visualization Script

Let your eyes shut gently. You may find that rotating your eyeballs upward slightly and inward, looking toward the center of your forehead with your eyes gently closed, helps you to relax more quickly. The important thing to do is to close your eyes, because you are about to shut out the world and start a voyage inward. Relaxation is the key to getting the most out of visualization. Take a deep, slow breath.

Now try to involve all of your senses. For example, try to visualize a piece of watermelon. Rather than just creating a visual picture in your mind, visualizing means hearing the crunch when you bite into it; feeling the cool, watery juice dripping onto your fingers and hands; smelling the unique odor; seeing the bright pink color contrasted against the black, shiny seeds; and finally tasting the sweet meat of the watermelon itself.

You can practice using all your senses by trying some of these brief visualization exercises.

For sight images, imagine a black circle on a white background. Now change the color of the circle to red. Let the circle fade until it becomes a dull pink. Now let it fade out entirely. (Reader: pause for ten seconds.)

For sound images, close your eyes and allow all shapes and colors to go away, imagining a dense, gray fog. Now imagine you that hear a phone ringing. Let it ring five times, then stop. (Reader: pause for five seconds.) *Now hear a car horn in the distance or a bird chirping overhead. Add some city sounds of construction or a fire engine in the distance. Now hear your parent saying your name in a loving tone.* (Reader: pause for ten seconds.)

For touch images, close your eyes and block out all visual or auditory images. Imagine sitting on a blanket with your toes in warm sand, or touching soft fur as you pet a cat, or squishing suds in your hands. (Reader: pause for ten seconds.)

For smell images, close out all sights, sounds, and touch, and focus on smelling freshly baked bread, or salt air, or freshly cut grass, or coffee brewing in the next room. (Reader: pause for ten seconds.)

Now that you've explored the experience of your senses in these individual exercises, you are ready to travel to your safe place. (Reader: pause for fifteen seconds.)

(Note: begin the recording here when you feel you are getting good at the above exercises.)

Now you are going to go to your safe place. Take a nice slow, deep breath. Now put your palms gently over your closed eyes and gently brush your hands over your eyes and face. Place your hands at your sides and allow your body to become relaxed all over. You are about to allow yourself to privately enter your own special place that is peaceful, comfortable, and safe. You will fill your imagination of this place with rich detail. You will experience this place close up, looking off into the distance, and through all of your senses. You can also allow room for another person, such as your spouse, friend, or family member, to be with you in this place if you choose.

Your safe place may be at the end of a boardwalk leading to a beach. Sand is under your feet, the water is about twenty yards away, and seagulls, boats, and clouds are in the distance. You feel the coolness of the air as a cloud passes in front of the sun, and seagulls are calling to each other. The sun is shimmering on the waves continually rolling to the shore, and there are smells of food emanating from the boardwalk.

A different safe place might be a warm, wood-paneled den, with the smell of cinnamon buns baking in the oven in the kitchen. Through a window, you can see fields of tall, dried cornstalks, and there is a crackling fire in the fireplace. A set of candles emit the aroma of lavender, and there is cup of warm tea on the table for you.

You may have a different safe place than these two scenes. Take a few seconds to identify your safe place. It can be the beach or a warm house, or anywhere else. The point is that it is your place to go to. (Reader: pause for ten seconds now and pause briefly after each sentence during this next section.)

Close your eyes now and get totally comfortable. Walk slowly to your safe and quiet place. Let your mind take you there. Your place can be indoors or outdoors. But wherever it is, it is peaceful and safe. Picture letting your anxieties and worries pass. Look to the distance. What do you see? Create a visual image of what you see in the distance. What do you smell? What do you hear? Notice what is right in front of you. Reach out and touch it. How does it feel? Smell it. Listen for any pleasant sounds. Make the temperature comfortable. Be safe here. Look around for a special, private spot. Feel the ground or earth under your feet. What does it feel like? Look above you. What do you see? What do you hear? What do you smell?

Now walk a bit further and stop. Reach out and touch something lightly with your fingertips. What is the texture of the object you are touching? This is your special place, and nothing can harm or upset you here. You can come here and relax whenever you want. Stay in this safe and peaceful place for as long as you wish, allowing yourself to breathe slowly and deeply and become relaxed all over. (Reader: pause for ten seconds.)

Is there anyone else you wish to be with you? If so, imagine that person is now with you, also enjoying the peace and calm of your safe place. If not, that's fine—this is your vacation. (Reader: pause for fifteen seconds.)

Now slowly rise and leave your safe place by the same path or steps that you used to enter. Notice your surroundings. Say to yourself, I can relax here. This is my special place, and I can come here whenever I wish.

Now slowly open your eyes and get used to your surroundings, but bring back with you the nice feelings of relaxation.

TRACK YOUR PROGRESS

As with the relaxation tools, it's a good idea to notice how tense you are before and after each session (use the SUDS approach as described in chapter 14). You can make notes in your journal each time you practice the exercise to track your progress. It's normal for your mind to occasionally wander during visualization. This will happen less often as you practice more. Don't be discouraged if you don't feel calm or relaxed after one or two attempts. The more you practice, the better this technique will work. As with physical exercise, the benefits will be evident after continued use, because you will have conditioned your mind to create a calm mental and physical state.

18

Visualization Tool:
Visualizing Success

Visualization is the conscious and intentional creation of impressions that use all five senses (seeing, hearing, smelling, touching, and tasting) for the purpose of changing yourself in some way. There are different reasons people use visualization, but the purpose of the "Visualizing Success" tool is to help you reach personal goals. We developed this tool several years ago and have found it to be very effective in initially motivating people to try to work toward a goal as well as in helping them to remain on such a path (Nezu et al. 1998).

VISUALIZATION IS EFFECTIVE

Five minutes of visualization can do more to help you realize your goals than any amount of worry or negative thinking. Several sessions a day can make a difference in helping you reach your goals, learn new skills, and change bad habits. This tool helps you to use your imagination and create a vision of a future that you can actually achieve.

Visualization can be a very effective tool for changing aspects of your life as well as for setting new goals. Goals can include changing your behavior, improving your relationships with family and friends, achieving professional and academic dreams, and improving sports performance. They can also include health goals (such as reducing smoking, increasing exercise, or changing diet), spiritual goals (such as personal growth), or leisure goals (such as going on more vacations).

VISUALIZING SUCCESS

Follow the visualization lessons below in order, beginning with lesson 1. Note that for lesson 4, you should ask a friend or family member with a calming voice to make a recording of the visualization script. This way, you will have your own visualization tape that you can use over and over again.

Move on to the next visualization lesson when you are ready. You can take any-where from one day to several weeks to get through the eight lessons. If you decide to take some time with any one of the lessons, just make sure to practice the visualization exercise that is described in that lesson at least once each day.

Lesson 1: Develop a specific visual picture of the future

Many times, people set personal goals that are too vague and cloudy. For example, if your goal is to improve your health, what is your visual picture of this goal? Do you see yourself eating three well-balanced meals a day? Do you picture yourself completing five push-ups and running two miles? Do you picture yourself with a blood pressure of 120 over 75, smoke free, or meditating in the park? Do you picture playing catch with your grandchildren in the park? Likewise, a goal for more financial security might include increasing your savings to a certain amount, starting a retirement plan, or picturing yourself in your own apartment.

It is very important that you develop your visualization of the future in very specific and concrete mental pictures. Try it out right now. Describe the mental picture of what you wish to accomplish and write down a description of that picture. For example, a person who wants to learn how to scuba dive might picture himself in warm, clear water, wearing a wet suit and scuba gear, slowly following the path of a beautiful fish. He approaches the surface with a sense of enjoyment and satisfaction. Later, he pictures himself sitting in the warm sun on the deck of the boat, sharing the experience with friends.

Lesson 2: Break down your visual picture of the future into a series of snapshots

It is important to have both short- and long-term goals to visualize. If your long-range visualization is seeing yourself smoke free and walking one mile each day, make a series of visual images that are steps to this goal. For example, you might have a short-range goal of cutting out smoking while on the telephone and walking at least two blocks each day. The next step might include no smoking after meals and walking five blocks a day, and so on. Practice visualizing images of both short- and long-term goals.

Lesson 3: Make sure your goals are about you

Remember to visualize your goals in terms of things that you can accomplish. You can only make changes in yourself. For example, if your overall goal is to improve your marriage, goals such as *my husband will not complain so much, my wife will not drink too much,* or *my husband will find me attractive* may not be reachable because they are not in your control. However, *I will be more patient, I will communicate my concerns and disagreement with her behavior more effectively,* or *I will feel more confident about the way I look* are goals that can be achieved because they involve things that you have control over. In the same way, goals involving physical or athletic accomplishments should be focused on improving *your* performance, not simply winning a game or an event. Winning involves other players' performances—something over which you have no control. When you define your goals in terms of yourself, your goals are actually reachable.

Lesson 4: Remove the barriers to your goals through visualization

In this lesson, you will travel, in your imagination, to the future and visit yourself five years from now. In this "daydream," remember that anything goes, so picture it just the way you want it to be. You will look around at your possessions, notice your accomplishments, see who you are with, be aware of how you spend your leisure time, and so on. Remember, it is a good idea to have a friend or family member with a calming voice record the script.

To prepare yourself to practice visualization, find a comfortable place to sit or lie down. Remember to loosen your clothing, remove glasses or contact lenses, and lower the lights. A single session will take about ten to fifteen minutes to complete. Remember that visualization becomes more effective through continued practice.

Use affirmations to state your intention to yourself when you begin the visualization. Examples include:

- *I will experience success in my mind.*

- *I have peace within myself.*

- *A goal is a possible future.*

- *If I can dream it, I can do it!*

- *I can put distractions aside for now.*

Script for Visualizing Success

(Reader: read softly and slowly, pausing between sentences throughout.)

Close your eyes and relax. Let go of any tension in your body. Now go to a safe and tranquil place in your mind—a special, outdoor place. Look around. Take note of what you see nearby as well as in the distance. Describe the scene silently to yourself. Now look for a path. This is your path toward the future. Notice a tree stump or log across the path. Imagine that this piece of wood is going to make it difficult for you to walk down the path. This piece of wood is your own hesitation or fear of changing and walking toward your goals. Step over it. Step over this log and visualize overcoming your hesitation, overcoming your fears.

Now, as you walk along the path, you come to the bottom of a steep hill. This hill is your own doubts about yourself. Slowly keep walking up the hill, even though you are not absolutely sure of what you will find at the top of the hill. With each step, begin to let yourself become more confident that you will reach your goals. (Reader: pause for five seconds.)

When you reach the top, you walk through a dark forest of trees that block out the sunlight. This forest represents all the obstacles that block you from seeing your final goals: interference from others, day-to-day problems that keep you from working on your goals, or your own fears that you don't deserve what you want. However, you push past the trees to a clearing, and you are now in a sunny field. You can see your home in the distance. This is your home five or ten years in the future. (Reader: pause for five seconds.)

Go into your home and look around. What do you see? How many rooms are there? How are they decorated? What things do you own? What pictures or photographs do you see? (Reader: pause for five seconds.) *Look at yourself in the mirror. What do you look like? What are you wearing?* (Reader: pause for five seconds.) *Watch as your family comes in. How do they treat each other? Listen to yourself as you imagine yourself to be five years older. Listen to yourself as you talk to people or make phone calls. What do you say?* (Reader: pause for five seconds.) *Follow yourself to work or school. What are your achievements? What are your activities?* (Reader: pause for five seconds.) *Watch yourself at leisure. What are you doing? For example, maybe you're watching TV, driving a racecar, sailing, fishing, or listening to classical music.* (Reader: pause for five seconds.)

Now ask yourself how you feel. Look back over your life of the last five years. What are you especially glad that you had the chance to experience? What are you most proud of? Maybe you gave a successful speech, you ran a marathon, you gained several good friends, you raised self-confident children, or people knew that they could count on you. Anything is possible. Remember to visualize what you hope and wish to be in the future, not what is going on now. (Reader: pause for five seconds.)

When you have finished exploring, let your images fade away and come back to the present, the here and now. Open your eyes, and while the images are still fresh in your mind, pick one or two major goals for your future and write down the details and the specific visual images that come to mind.

Lesson 5: Write down your five-year goal

Choose just one image from the previous visualization exercise and write down your five-year goal. It could be a personal, physical, career, family, or social goal. Remember to be very specific and concrete.

Lesson 6: Break down your goal into one-year goals

Look at the goal again and break it down into one-year goals—one goal for each year. These would be smaller steps leading to your larger goal. Write these down.

Lesson 7: Break your first-year goal into smaller steps

Now look at the *first* one-year goal and break it down into even smaller steps to reach over the course of a year. Write these down. Once again, remember to be very concrete and specific.

Lesson 8: Create a daily visualization

Create a visualization you can use every day to help you accomplish the steps toward these goals. In your imagination, picture yourself successfully carrying out the steps for your immediate goals. For example, one young woman we counseled pictured herself exercising two days per week for the next four months. She visualized herself in her workout clothes, imagining that she would experience a sense of pride in arranging for enough time to spend at the gym. She imagined her favorite music playing on her personal stereo, and she visualized her body feeling strong and the perspiration dripping off her skin. Every time she visualized this sequence, she made a stronger commitment to do it. After each workout, she found herself believing her visualizations and trusting herself to meet her goals. These visualization exercises helped her reach her goals.

We taught a male cardiac patient to visualize improving his performance as a high school basketball coach. He visualized going to the library once a week to borrow books about the sport and once a month watching films of good coaches at work. He pictured himself helping new players to develop their skills and increasing their motivation to do their best by really listening and reaching out to them when discussing team strategies. He, too, was able to reach his goals by using this tool.

As you reach each goal that you have visualized, begin daily visualizations of the next step in your series of goals, leading finally up to your one-year goal. After that, develop a series of visualization steps toward the next year's goal.

In general, use the basic strategy of visualizing goals for the future in order to develop a road map of steps that you need to take to achieve such goals, whether those steps involve solving a particular stressful problem at present, reaching toward a goal that takes only a week to accomplish, or going for something that involves a much longer time. In developing such road maps, write down overall goals as well as smaller steps leading to these goals. Visualize reaching each step, then go for it!

FINAL THOUGHTS

Sometimes people set unrealistic initial goals or set goals that depend on other people. If this happens to you, choose smaller goals that are reachable in a short period of time and be sure your goals are based on changes that are yours to make. You may find it very helpful to ask other people for support and encouragement. See chapter 19, "Getting Social Support," for ideas. In addition, if you are experiencing difficulties with obstacles or problems that block you from reaching your goals, refer to chapter 13, "Solving Stressful Problems."

19

Interpersonal Tool: Getting Social Support

Since the earliest times in history, people who stood together and supported each other have had a better chance of survival. This is as true today as it was in older times. And this is true not only for physical survival; social support is important to psychological and emotional survival as well. Scientific studies have shown that there is a very strong link between social support and psychological, emotional, and physical well-being (Manne 2003).

SOCIAL SUPPORT IS IMPORTANT TO YOUR HEALTH

Social support usually refers to having a variety of social contacts who are available as potential emotional and practical resources for your benefit. A positive social contact can be any relationship in which you experience pleasure, respect, understanding, help, companionship, stimulation, or any other positive human experience. The idea of social support can even be extended to animals or pets, which often provide companionship, comfort, and a sense of being needed. In essence, social support can help individuals cope more effectively with stress (Antonucci, Lansford, and Ajrouch 2000).

Although most people would think of this idea as common sense, there is a lot of psychological and medical research that demonstrates that people who have good social support tend to have a better overall quality of life and may actually live longer (Wills 1998). On the other hand, people who tend to be very isolated and distant from others often experience harmful effects, including loneliness, mental and emotional problems, and worsening of physical problems.

Here are some reasons social support may be beneficial to your health:

- People who know that others care often try to take better care of themselves. This can include doing things like maintaining good eating habits, exercising, and not smoking or drinking too much.

- People who have someone to turn to have a chance to vent and talk about bad experiences and negative feelings. When people do not have someone to talk to, they sometimes try to block out emotions or turn to drugs, alcohol, or other high-risk behaviors as a way of dealing with their problems.

- When receiving comfort, love, understanding, and care, people actually experience important biochemical and hormonal changes that may help the body (for example, the immune system) stay healthy.

- Other people can provide needed advice and guidance with problems. They can also help you reach your goals. They can be mentors, advisors, and colleagues.

Are All Social Relationships Good for Your Health?

As you may have guessed, there is also a negative side to social connections. All the positive effects of social support are based upon positive social support. A good marriage, for example, can contribute to good health, but a bad marriage can be very stressful and can actually work against your health. All the reasons above have the reverse effect when the social connection is stressful because the interaction is abusive, critical, angry, selfish, burdensome, or frustrating. If a current relationship is negative for you, refer to chapter 13, "Solving Stressful Problems," for coping strategies.

SOCIAL SUPPORT AND HEART DISEASE

Positive social support has been linked to both lower systolic blood pressure and lower diastolic blood pressure (Manne 2003). Moreover, inadequate social support has been associated with higher levels of mortality from coronary heart disease. The effect of poor social support as a risk factor is equal to that of smoking (Stoney 1998). Vogt and colleagues (1992), following a group of patients in a health maintenance organization for fifteen years, found that individuals who reported a wide range of social contacts were less likely to have a heart attack as compared to those with less social support, even after controlling for the presence of other medical problems such as obesity and diabetes.

Further, social support has been found to affect the outcome of cardiac rehabilitation not only directly but also indirectly, as it tends to reduce depression, leading to improved cardiac functioning (Shen, McCreary, and Myers 2004). Psychosocial interventions or counseling programs geared to provide emotional and social support have been found to be effective in significantly reducing the likelihood of a recurrence of heart attacks (Frasure-Smith and Prince 1985).

Given these significant links between social support and cardiovascular disease, this tool can be effective in helping to foster your own heart health.

GETTING STARTED

Some people express hesitation when we describe this strategy. If you have concerns, pay close attention to the following.

The purpose of this tool is to help you increase your positive social support. Don't wait for other people to make the first move. Your part in using this tool is to be creative in making sure that you get the social support you need.

In counseling heart patients to seek additional social support, we have frequently been asked, "If I have to ask for it, is it still social support?" Our answer is yes. Some people think that you shouldn't have to ask another person for companionship, support, or time together, because if other people wanted to be with you, they would ask you. However, if everyone felt this way, no one would ever ask anybody!

We have also frequently been asked another question: "If I ask for support and get turned down, won't it make things worse?" Our answer is no—unless you focus on getting turned down and give up. Some people are afraid they will be turned down if they invite someone out or suggest getting together. While this may happen, the odds are in your favor that you will get a positive response from most people. If you ask five people for companionship or support and two of them turn you down, that means that you will actually get support from three of those five people. Even with the rejections, wouldn't you rather be receiving more support and companionship than you have right now?

GETTING SOCIAL SUPPORT

We hope you now feel more motivated and prepared to seek additional social support. These steps will guide you through the process.

Step 1: List possible sources of support

Make a list of people who already provide or could provide positive companionship for you. Be creative when making this list and make sure that you include friends, neighbors, relatives, people from work or school, or people you encounter in your daily activities like shopping, going to the dry cleaner or the bank, or getting gas. Also include those who are members of the same community organizations you belong to, such as a charity, library, musical society, church, or political group.

Don't worry about any obstacles in the way, such as how busy these people are, how far away they live, how well you know them, or how long it's been since you have talked to them. Your first goal is make the longest list you can. Remember that telephone calls are often easier to arrange than visits. If there are people you enjoy talking to on the phone, be sure to include them on the list.

Pets and animals are another kind of social support. Consider opportunities to spend more time with animals you enjoy. For example, consider getting a pet, visiting someone with a pet you enjoy, going to the zoo, working at the animal shelter, volunteering at an animal clinic or veterinary office, or visiting the aquarium.

If you have difficulty coming up with a comprehensive list, use the brainstorming rules in chapter 13 to help you be more creative. You can also use this tool later if you encounter practical problems related to getting together with a potential friend (for example, differing schedules).

Step 2: List the benefits to both of you

Decide how you will make your interaction pleasant for both of you. Think about the visit from the other person's point of view as well as your own. Next to each name, write down why you would like to see that person and also what that person might enjoy about the visit with you.

Here are some examples.

- "My friend Jane works for a computer software company. She would probably like giving me advice about software programs for learning a foreign language. I would enjoy getting a software program to learn French."

- "My brother is very busy and never has time to cook anymore. I'll invite him over and get all the ingredients ready for his famous chili and ask him to make it together for dinner."

- "The people from the church are always asking for help with the blood drive. If I help, I'll meet new people and feel needed, and the church will get free help."

Step 3: Commit to at least one new social event in the next week

Now choose at least one activity from your list to do this coming week. Identify a person, group, pet, or activity (for example, joining a bowling team or church choir) that would represent an increase in your social support. For the next month, try to plan at least one social event each week as a means of improving your positive social support.

If you are having difficulty thinking about what to do with a friend, go to the list of positive experiences at the end of chapter 11.

Step 4: Remove negative social contacts from your list

Now go back over the list, this time looking for people who represent stress rather than a positive experience. For example, you may have a neighbor or relative who is always the center of attention and shows little concern for others. This is a person who is bound to disappoint you. Take such people off your list and politely decline their invitations. However, if you feel that a relationship is worth fighting for, then use the problem-solving strategies in chapter 13 to develop a plan to improve the relationship.

FINAL THOUGHTS

Social support can come from a positive relationship with another person, group, or even a pet. Positive social support can be beneficial to your emotional and physical health. Remember, not all social relationships are good for your health. Try to avoid those that are especially stressful. Think creatively of all the different people and groups that might be potential sources of social support. Take at least one step to increase your social support network each week for a month.

20

Spirituality Tool: Awakening Your Spirituality

Because all of the other chapters in this book address issues of the mind and body, we want to ensure that we also address the spirit. The majority of people in the world, including the United States, indicate that they endorse some type of religious or spiritual belief system (Koenig 1997). Given this, we feel it is important to address the spiritual issues related to heart health. We realize this chapter may not be relevant for you. However, we wish to provide a variety of tools—including ones based on spirituality and faith—from which you can choose.

Each person's spiritual experiences are unique, private, and internal. Spirituality is an individual's view of the world that is inward focused, because through spirituality, people are able to be in touch with themselves and their inner energy. It is also outward focused, because through a spiritual perspective, people are able to recognize the connection they have with each other as well as with something greater than themselves. For some people, this something greater is represented by a higher power, such as God, Allah, or Buddha. For others, the connection to something greater may be found in the cosmos, universe, multiple deities, or the sanctity of nature, as in the Japanese Shinto philosophy.

HOW SPIRITUALITY IS DIFFERENT THAN RELIGION

Spirituality does not necessarily involve a formal religion, although for many people, religious faith is a central part of their spirituality. Religion provides the social and cultural part of spiritual experience. For example, each religion has its own practices, including traditions, services, and ritual activities, as well as scriptures, stories, and doctrines. Examples include studying the Torah, singing Christian hymns, making a Catholic confession, the telling of Native American myths and legends, or the ecstatic dancing of a Muslim dervish. Spirituality is the more individual, subjective experience people have when they engage in a personal search for answers to ultimate life questions, such as the meaning of life and its association to that which is sacred or transcendent.

You do not need to have a specific religion in order to be spiritual. A review of a wide range of traditional and contemporary approaches to spirituality reveals that there are common messages and practices across both religious and nonreligious spiritual philosophies. These include messages of love, acceptance, and compassion and practices of meditation, singing, chanting, and congregation with people who share common beliefs.

SPIRITUAL AWARENESS AND HEALTH

People who are spiritually aware see themselves as having an inner essence or energy (some use the word "soul") that is connected to others. As such, they are equal in worth and importance to all others. This view can serve to awaken self-esteem, tolerance, and hopefulness. In addition, reviews of scientific research show that there is a strong association between spirituality and improved health outcomes. For example, a patient's spirituality can enhance coping and recovery from illness (Mueller, Plevak, and Rummans 2001). A spiritual focus can decrease anxiety and depression, improve immune functioning, and increase experiences of joy, enthusiasm, and goodwill (Goleman 2003).

With regard to cardiovascular health, Morris (2001) found that spiritual well-being was significantly correlated with improved coronary heart disease among a group of patients who participated in the original Ornish Lifestyle Heart Trial, which included meditation. In addition, King and colleagues (2001) found a significant association between higher religious attendance and lowered risk for cardiovascular disease. Among older adults living in community settings, Koenig and colleagues (1998) found that those who frequently attended religious services had lower blood pressure than those who attended infrequently. Private religious activity, such as prayer, meditation, or scripture reading, was also strongly associated with lowered blood pressure. Certain religious or spiritual rituals have been found to have a positive effect on cardiovascular health. Specifically, recitation of rosary prayers or yoga mantras was found to slow breathing rate, lower both systolic and diastolic blood pressure, and increase blood flow in the brain (Bernardi et al. 2001).

CULTIVATING SPIRITUAL AWARENESS

Right now, try an experiment to tap into your spirituality. Reflect back to a moment when you were completely delighted and grateful to be alive, even for an instant. Maybe you saw your baby smile for the first time, watched a sunset, engaged in an act of aid or compassion for another, experienced gratitude for a delicious food when you were hungry, or felt a cold, crisp autumn wind on your face. Write down a brief description of the experience in your journal now.

Describe the subjective feeling you had during this experience. If you are like most people, you would say that this was a time when you were awakened to the joy of living—even if just for a moment, before your mind had a chance to wander and worry about other things. Increasing your spiritual awareness can help you to increase your appreciation of life's spiritual moments when you are facing the day-to-day stresses of life.

When people are spiritually aware, their experience is less hindered by worry or regret, and they are more likely to set goals for change, more motivated to put their values into practice, and more effective at solving day-to-day problems (Nezu and Nezu 2003). Specific techniques for increasing spiritual awareness are designed to remove the barriers of a busy mind that focuses on negative self-talk. These can be powerful tools in and of themselves as a means of decreasing anxiety and increasing your sense of well-being and calmness. Moreover, such techniques can help you to step back and observe your often self-destructive thinking habits. As a result, spirituality can help you to put into practice many of the other tools in this book that focus on decreasing negative self-talk and anxious worry.

In this chapter, we provide specific strategies to help foster your spiritual awareness. The first tool, *mindfulness meditation,* involves learning how to stay in the present moment, becoming more aware of your surroundings while observing your internal experiences without judgment or evaluation. This tool can also help you to be more appreciative of the transient nature of reality and to accept such changes. Being able to stay in the present, accept change, and reduce internal judgment can set into motion a series of physical and biochemical changes that can have significant positive effects on your cardiovascular system and your immune system. It is difficult to say just how much the positive cardiovascular effects of spirituality are due to decreased anxiety and depression, increased positive emotional experiences, or direct physiological changes over time, but all of these pathways to improved well-being have been proposed.

MINDFULNESS MEDITATION

Mindfulness refers to a centuries-old meditative practice that has been an integral part of spiritual training in various Eastern religious faiths, including Buddhism. It has been a strong aspect of some mystic Christian contemplative traditions as well. Mindfulness has been described as a state of nonjudgmental awareness—essentially the ability, through practice, to be fully aware of a situation without having to add anything to it and without judging what you are experiencing. Similar in practice to some of the relaxation tools in this book, mindfulness allows you to more fully experience what is happening in the present moment (that is, your breathing, your bodily sensations, your immediate environment, your movement, your present activity) without getting caught up in thoughts or emotional reactions. This ability then helps you to regulate your own responses to day-to-day stressors.

Mindfulness meditation can help you cope with a stressful event by approaching the situation mindfully, simply responding to it rather than automatically reacting to it in ways that have been maladaptive or destructive in the past. Research continues to find this approach to be effective for a variety of human problems. Alan Marlatt, a prominent behavioral psychologist, has found mindfulness meditation to be helpful in the treatment of addictions, including excessive drinking and alcoholism (Marlatt and Kristeller 1999). Jon Kabat-Zinn, a pioneer in the application of this approach in medicine, found mindfulness meditation to be effective in reducing chronic pain (Kabat-Zinn, Lipworth, and Burney 1985). Other researchers have proposed that mindfulness is helpful in the treatment of depression (Teasdale et al. 2000) and self-destructive behavior (Dimidjian and Linehan 2003).

With regard to heart health, meditation techniques have been found to have significant beneficial effects on blood pressure and cholesterol levels (Walton et al. 2002). Meditation has also been found to improve heart rate variability (Barnes, Treiber, and Davis 2001) as well as decrease exercise-induced myocardial ischemia in patients with coronary artery disease (Zamarra et al. 1996). It has also been found to lower serum cortisol, diastolic blood pressure, systolic blood pressure, and pulse rate (Sudsuang, Chentanez, and Veluvan 1991).

An important aspect of mindfulness meditation is the idea of distancing yourself from your experiences. As an independent observer or onlooker, you pay close attention to your thoughts and feelings as they occur in the present moment, but you attempt to separate these thoughts and feelings from your inner self. In other words, you can eventually, through this process, come to understand that you are not your thoughts and you are not your feelings. In this way, you can observe thoughts and feelings—including negative ones—as you experience them, while realizing that you don't have to allow these thoughts and feelings to force you to act in a certain way. As such, the thought *I feel so stupid today for getting nervous* is just a thought. You can note it, observe it, and even see it pass by. But most importantly, you don't have to *react* to such a thought as if it is the universal truth and then feel bad about yourself. You can simply acknowledge, with detached acceptance, that you had a thought. The thought doesn't own you, nor does it define you—it's just a thought.

We have found that the metaphor of looking at movies of yourself or hearing recordings of your voice can be a useful way to help you become a detached observer. Seeing a movie of yourself allows you to see yourself from outside of your own body. You are actually seeing yourself say and do things—but it really isn't you. If you can refrain from evaluating these actions and instead simply note that you are engaged in them, then you can begin to see your thoughts and feelings from a distance. If you have ever taken any home movies, go look at them now and try to simply observe yourself. Try to observe yourself without any judgments, being more accepting and forgiving of any actions about which you previously would have felt embarrassed (or even proud). Simply observe—don't judge.

GETTING DISTANCE FROM YOUR INTERNAL JUDGE

This tool is designed to help release you from your mind's tendency to fill up with thoughts of guilt, resentment of the past, or worry about the future; feelings of pride; or perceptions of superiority. Any of these types of thoughts can only take you away from experiencing the present moment.

Over the next few minutes, try this brief exercise. Close your eyes, clear your mind, and just observe the first thought of which you are conscious. You may actually be thinking, *What is the first thought that comes into my mind?* It may take a few seconds or several minutes. What was the thought? It may have been a comment on the exercise, such as *This seems silly, I wonder if I'm doing this correctly,* or *I can't take time to do this now—I'm wasting time!* Before your first thought, you were in the present and away from your busy mind.

This exercise is designed to bring home several important points about how to practice mindfulness meditation.

- As long as you are in a state of intense presence, you are free of thought. You are still, your mind is calm, yet you remain highly alert.

- The instant your conscious attention slips a bit, a thought rushes in that takes you away from the moment.

- For the brief time that you had a clear mind, as well as the time you were observing a thought that popped into your head, you were in the moment, aware of your thought, waiting for it, and able to notice it without evaluation, accepting whatever was there. *This, essentially, is the definition of mindfulness.*

- The thought you experienced probably contained some kind of critique, worry, instruction, memory, daydream, or positive or negative judgment about yourself. This is how your mind has generally learned to pull you away from the moment.

■   If you are able to observe your mind "speaking" or transmitting a thought, remember that you are not your mind. Your mind is essentially a tool that can be used to help connect you with your true inner self. Alternatively, it can work against you and lead you to chronically avoid or ignore the precious experience that is your life. By learning to separate and disengage your mind's thinking habits from who you are, you will become more aware of your own purpose and potential as well as the beauty that exists in the world.

Mindfulness Can Help You Unlearn Old Thinking Habits

This meditation tool is designed to help you develop your mindfulness skills. Over the years, you may have learned to automatically respond to your mind telling you that you must gain approval from others; avoid unpleasant thoughts, feelings, or memories; and ignore who you really are. Paradoxically, the reason for this involves the way in which the brain works. Human beings have a uniquely sophisticated way of processing information through words that allows us to be capable of great insights and innovations. At the same time, this very complex type of information processing is designed to help us avoid danger in order to survive. This can be very useful when you are confronted with a physically dangerous situation and your mind uses all of its processing abilities to put information together to warn you of the danger.

This same ability, however, can be useless and destructive when it puts information together to warn you of nondeadly consequences. Day-to-day examples of the mind warning you of this type of "danger" include embarrassment, fear of the unknown, confusion, hostility, and need for approval. Responding to such thinking habits can take you away from being spiritually present in a meaningful life moment. Meditation connects you with your inner energies or life force and helps you stop shutting yourself off from your potential. Ultimately, by learning to focus more on the here and now, you can realign yourself with your true path—the path to inner peace.

MINDFULNESS BREATHING MEDITATION

Now you're ready to learn how to meditate in a mindful manner. The best time to practice this meditation tool may be in the early morning, just after awakening. You have had some rest and have not yet turned on the television or radio to begin the bombardment of messages to your mind. However, you can choose any place or time to engage in mindful breathing: at your office, before retiring for the night, in your car while waiting to pick up your children, or even while waiting for a red light to change.

You may practice this meditation with your eyes open or closed. Some people find it easier to tune in to their breathing when their eyes are closed. However, this would not be advisable in certain situations, such as driving or walking across a busy street. Initially, plan on about ten minutes to engage in this mindfulness breathing meditation exercise. You can extend the time after you have practiced a bit. You may wish to record the following instructions so you don't have to remember them. These instructions are adapted from the mindfulness training developed by Jon Kabat-Zinn (1995). If you find the technique helpful, you may want to supplement these instructions with recordings that are commercially available.

Begin by feeling your breath. Do not think about it—feel it come in.

Notice how it stops, it reverses, then it flows out.

There is no special way to breathe. Any way you breathe is natural; it is your life force.

Think of your breath like a rising wave: it happens on its own. Just stay with that. Be mindful of the breath in your own body.

Your mind is not going to want to stay on the breath for very long. When you drop your focus on your breathing, just let the mind go off—but let it also come back.

Leave your body still.

Feel the breath.

Breathe in . . . breathe out.

As you breathe in, focus on the in-breath. You are accepting life.

As you exhale, focus on the out-breath. You are giving life.

Ride the breath.

Flow with the breath.

Feel it in your nostrils.

Feel your abdomen rise and fall. (If you like, place your hands on your belly to feel the flow of your breath.)

Rest your mind on the simple, regular, calming wave of breathing that your body is experiencing.

Notice the sensation in your nostrils, abdomen, and shoulders.

Notice any thoughts that bubble up to the surface of the mind. Notice them and simply let them go. Remember that these thoughts are not you—you are not defined by your thoughts.

Settle in the present moment. Be aware of actual moment-to-moment happenings: a slight pain in your shoulder, an itch on your arm, or various sounds, such as a train passing by, the wind rustling through the trees, or people's voices.

Let your concentration deepen.

Don't try to suppress your perceptions, feelings, or awareness—simply notice what is happening and then let it dissolve as a new moment begins.

Stay awake, even if your eyes are closed. Remain alert. Pay attention.

Breathe in . . . breathe out. Stay focused.

Let go of each breath. Let go of each thought—don't hang on.

Note your thoughts. Notice them and let them go. With each breath, let go of any thoughts a little bit more. Let them simply pass by.

Notice where your mind is when it's not on your breathing.

Make no judgment, just notice where it is and come back to the breath.

Allow each moment to be fresh and new.

After you engage in several practice sessions, it is likely that you will have experienced several moments in which you were able to let the noise of your mind fade in the background and experience the present moment. Try to practice this tool at least once a day for a week or two. We suggest that you consider practicing this tool once a week for the rest of your life.

After each session, write down any impressions you have in your journal: whether you enjoyed it, whether you experienced an increase in your ability to be in the moment and notice things you have learned to say to yourself that get in the way of a peaceful mind. Over time, these observations can provide meaningful insight concerning your mindfulness practice.

Mindfulness as a Way of Life

As we indicated when we first introduced the concept of mindfulness, sitting still or lying down is not a requirement for a meditation experience. Activities and tasks such as walking, gardening, cooking, painting, or even eating can be accomplished in a mindful manner that keeps you focused in the present. The benefit you receive from exercising your mindfulness skills during simple tasks is that you are able to consciously capture the full experience of your day-to-day activities as important and valuable. For example, consider how you might thoughtlessly eat a piece of fruit during the day. Now imagine taking a moment to appreciate the texture, smell, and availability of the fruit you are holding, and imagine noticing the taste and juiciness as you slowly savor it. Mindfulness provides a whole new way to focus your attention on simple activities throughout the day. The following instructions will help you turn a twenty-minute walk—which you can take in the morning, at lunchtime, or in the evening after work—into a spiritual and mindful experience to help your heart.

A MINDFUL WALK

Allow yourself at least twenty minutes to take this type of walk. This is not a walk for physical exercise, and you can feel free to sit down at any time. The importance of this exercise is that you will have an opportunity to practice a walking meditation. Try taking such a walk at least once a week—perhaps for the rest of your life.

Begin by engaging in mindful breathing, which you learned in the previous exercise.

As you breathe in, be aware that you are receiving life.

As you exhale, be aware that you are giving something back to the world.

Stay in the present.

Clear all thoughts of the past or future.

Stay in touch with your breathing.

As any thoughts come to mind, simply observe them and let them pass.

Let any of these thoughts go and refocus on the present.

The purpose is to be present and aware of your breathing and walking.

Be aware of your feet as you walk, one foot in front of the other.

Walk gently on the earth. Be aware that with every step, you are placing your footprint on the earth.

You can coordinate your breathing with your steps by taking an in-breath every few steps, followed by an out-breath every few steps. You may quietly whisper "in" and "out" to yourself as you go along your path.

Notice how your feet and legs are able to make each step the correct length.

Be aware of all other sights, smells, and life in your surroundings: the car horns, the birds, the traffic noises, the leaves on a tree, the blades of grass, the concrete walkway, the park bench, or the mall parking lot.

Notice that everything you see is imperfect and impermanent. The tree's bark has cracks in it indicating its age or the conditions under which it grew.

As you walk along a concrete path, you may notice that it is cracked or covered with leaves, debris, or animal droppings.

Be aware of people. Notice how imperfect yet beautiful they are.

Visualize how you are connected to each person in some way or they to each other.

Be aware of the life and energy that is around you—the people, plants, and animals.

What is present in your surroundings that you cannot see? Perhaps a squirrel that darts behind a tree, the pain experienced by an aging woman who crosses the street with her cane, or the bulbs of spring flowers that are still under the frozen ground. Be aware that even though you may be aware of all that you observe, there are things present that you cannot see with your eyes.

As you return from your walk, be aware of all those things that you may have missed on previous walks. Make a commitment to become more mindful as you go through each day in order that you may connect with your true inner self and the true inner selves of others.

The tools to increase spiritual awareness thus far have focused on mindfulness meditation to calm and focus your mind. Now we'll move on to another tool to strengthen your spirituality by cultivating a sense of gratitude.

THE BENEFITS OF A GRATEFUL DISPOSITION

The second spirituality tool we provide in this chapter involves increasing your ability to be grateful. Enhancing your capacity to experience gratitude can help to decrease your experience of anger and hostility. Practically speaking, gratitude is incompatible with these negative emotional states. Although you may go back and forth between the two, it is impossible to experience gratitude and anger at the same moment. Therefore, the more you become aware of gratitude through conscious practice, the more you will free yourself from hostile thoughts and angry reactions. This can have enormous benefits to your physical and emotional well-being. Gratitude researchers Emmons and McCullough (2003), for example, recently found that helping individuals to "focus more on their blessings" led to more positive and optimistic appraisals of their lives, increased physical exercise, fewer physical symptoms, improved mood, more sleep, improved sleep quality, and an enhanced sense of connectedness to others.

Accepting Life's Gifts with Gratitude

With a little help and guidance, you can learn to be more aware of the many gifts that you receive "free of charge" in life. Let's begin by taking a look at some of the gifts you have received but may have ignored over the past week. We'll start you off by pointing out common gifts that people receive. You may want to jot down in your journal some of these free gifts that apply to you so you can remember to practice being grateful in the future. However, please don't stop with these, but add to your own inventory of free gifts for which you're grateful.

The gift of healing. This gift miraculously occurs when a cut on your finger or the bruise on your knee disappears after a few days. Consider for a moment the complicated array of biological and physiological miracles that occur every day to heal wounds, adapt your body to environmental changes, pump blood through your body to nourish vital organs, battle viral infections, and return your heart rate to normal after physical exercise. Have you let these gifts of healing go unrecognized?

The gift of work. Despite the daily hassles and stresses of your work, consider the millions of people in the world who have no gainful means of employment or recognition of their efforts. In addition, consider all the work you do—such as housecleaning, laundry, personal accounting, and walking the dog—for which you don't get paid. Your gratitude for the opportunity to finish a job, provide a service, or care for others is a gift. Your gratitude for such gifts will help to keep your emotions positive and help you manage the day-to-day stressors that you face.

The gifts of other people. Think about the people in your life now who have turned out to be wonderful and surprising gifts. We have spoken to many patients with heart disease, as well as other medical challenges, who indicated that their illness brought people into their lives for whom they were very grateful. This surely included doctors and nurses but also physical therapists, other patients, technicians, psychologists, and previous acquaintances who provided unexpected support, insights, and joy in their lives.

The gifts of nourishment. Imagine the possibilities for gratitude if you stop to notice the gifts you have that enable you to have access to clean water or healthy food. Have you recognized the gift of someone who cooks meals for you or your own ability to cook a meal? The next time you are shopping, take a moment to look at the choices you have in front of you in each section of the supermarket.

The gifts of education. Although many people become sidetracked with worry about attending the right schools or resentment over the costs of college, look at the opportunities for learning that you are given. In addition to the public education available to you, there are learning opportunities available through libraries, museums, radio, television, and public lectures that can fill an entire lifetime.

The gifts of transportation. Think about the gifts you have available to be able to drive a car, fly thousands of miles in just hours on an airplane, or ride in an air-conditioned bus.

PRACTICING GRATITUDE

Get out your journal once again and follow these instructions for practicing gratitude for the large and small gifts in your life. These may be gifts that you receive from others, through physical or environmental forces, or from a higher power.

Step 1: Find two things to be grateful for each day

Write down at least two things for which you were grateful during each day for one week. The way to identify the things for which you are grateful is to be on the lookout for even small moments in which you experience a surge of joy. If you find it difficult to limit yourself to two things, great! Don't feel that you have to stop at two. Remember that anything can qualify. For example, our own personal lists have included things as big as the support and love we give to each other, a chance to share moments with our children and grandchild, or seeing our patients grow stronger. These also include the small things, such as the chance to hear a great music CD, take a hot shower, taste good wine, feel the sun's warmth on our faces, smell the salt air, or take a walk. Remember to write down two things for each day. First describe the item or event for which you are grateful. Next, briefly describe *why* you are grateful. Remember that you don't have to physically experience the event—just thinking about it will qualify. For example, if you are reflecting on a shared moment with a friend or enjoying your vision of an upcoming holiday or event, your internal vision of the experience can serve as an important moment of gratitude.

Step 2: Review your list

At the end of the week, read over all of the things that you wrote down. Notice how at the moment you reexperience your gratitude, there is an absence of hostility, envy, anger, jealousy, or resentment.

Step 3: Use gratitude to counteract negative emotions

When you do experience hostility, envy, anger, jealousy, or resentment, or when you're just plain feeling sorry for yourself, take out your list and review all the things for which you are grateful. Allow yourself to focus on any one pleasant gift. Close your eyes, breathe deeply, and allow gratitude to fill your heart. Remember the words of the Buddhist teacher Thich Nhat Hanh: "When I have a toothache, I discover that not having a toothache is a wonderful thing. That is peace" (1999, 41).

FINAL THOUGHTS

As you use the tools in this chapter, remember that they provide only a small window or first step into the possibilities of the emotional, psychological, and physical benefits of becoming more aware of your inner self, of awakening your spirituality. We decided to focus on mindfulness and gratitude because they are particularly potent antidotes for anger, anxiety, and depression. If you keep an open mind, you can further explore your spirituality through various religious and nonreligious activities and practices available through books, tapes, organizations, and community activities. For more guidance, see our 2003 book, *Awakening Self-Esteem: Spiritual and Psychological Techniques to Enhance Your Well-Being* (New Harbinger Publications).

Feelings Test for Spouses and Others

Your spouse, family member, or friend has asked you to complete this questionnaire because you are someone who knows him or her well. Please be as honest as possible and answer each of the thirty-three questions in this questionnaire. If you are not certain, make the best guess possible, based on this person's behavior, what he or she generally says, or how he or she generally seems to feel. It is important to understand that even if you believe you might be hurting this person's feelings, by answering honestly, you are actually helping him or her change for the better. Simply circle yes or no based on your direct experience with this person.

Does this person . . .

1. act sad or down much of the day?   Yes   No

2. act tired and fatigued, like he or she has less energy than before?   Yes   No

3. often get upset at people who act superior?   Yes   No

4. continue to yell at people who wrong him or her (for example,   Yes   No
   cut in front on the grocery line) for several minutes after the
   event happens?

5. often appear out of breath when not exercising?   Yes   No

6. get very angry when he or she is the butt of a joke?   Yes   No

7. often express feelings of worthlessness or guilt?   Yes   No

8. frequently express feelings of fear or dread?   Yes   No

9. often have cold feet or hands?   Yes   No

10. often act hopeless and pessimistic?   Yes   No

11. often say things like, "What a jerk!"?   Yes   No

12. get angry at people who are rude?   Yes   No

13. have thoughts about harming himself or herself?   Yes   No

14. seem to have lost interest in activities that were once pleasurable?   Yes   No

15. frequently talk about feeling like his or her head is about to explode from anger?   Yes   No

16. act restless or mention having tight muscles?   Yes   No

17. have problems concentrating or making decisions?   Yes   No

18. get angry frequently?   Yes   No

19. frequently say things like, "Why doesn't that person just shut up?"   Yes   No

20. have problems with going to sleep, waking up in the middle of the night, or oversleeping?   Yes   No

21. have headaches, stomachaches, or other pains that are not connected to a medical problem?   Yes   No

22. react roughly to people who are annoying to him or her?   Yes   No

23. seem to have lost interest in sex?   Yes   No

24. sweat or perspire a lot?   Yes   No

25. often yell at someone but appear to forget why he or she originally got angry?   Yes   No

26. often have intrusive thoughts about a traumatic event that he or she experienced? Yes No?

27. often get angry at people who violate one of his or her basic beliefs, values, or principles? Yes No

28. appear to be afraid of the future? Yes No

29. often get angry when people are taking too long to do something (for example, taking too long at the post office counter, driving slowly)? Yes No

30. worry a lot about things in general? Yes No

31. experience dizziness or light-headedness? Yes No

32. seem to have lost or gained weight without really trying to? Yes No

33. seem to feel uncertain and uneasy about what is happening in his or her life? Yes No

References

Achterberg, J., B. Dossey, L. Kolkmeier, and A. A. Sheikh. 2003. Use of imagery in the treatment of cardiovascular disorders. In *Healing Images: The Role of Imagination in Health,* edited by A. A. Sheikh. Amityville, N.Y.: Baywood Publishing.

American Heart Association. 2004. Heart Disease and Stroke Statistics—2004 Update. www.americanheart.org.

Anda, R., D. Williamson, D. Jones, C. Macea, E. Eaker, A. Glassman, and J. Marks. 1993. Depressed affect, hopelessness, and the risk of ischemic heart disease in a cohort of U.S. adults. *Epidemiology* 4:285–94.

Antonucci, T. C., J. E. Lansford, and K. J. Ajrouch. 2000. Social support. In *Encyclopedia of Stress,* vol. 3, edited by G. Fink. New York: Academic Press.

Barefoot, J. C., and M. Schroll. 1996. Symptoms of depression, acute myocardial infarction, and total mortality in a community sample. *Circulation* 93:1976–80.

Barnes, V. A., F. A. Treiber, and H. Davis. 2001. Impact of Transcendental Meditation on cardiovascular function at rest and during acute stress in adolescents with high normal blood pressure. *Journal of Psychosomatic Research* 51:597–605.

Beck, A. T. 1976. *Cognitive Therapy and the Emotional Disorders.* New York: International Universities Press.

Beck, J. S. 1995. *Cognitive Therapy: Basics and Beyond.* New York: Guilford Press.

Berkman, L. F., L. Leo-Summers, and R. I. Horwitz. 1992. Emotional support and survival after myocardial infarction. A prospective, population-based study of the elderly. *Annals of Internal Medicine* 117:1003–9.

Bernardi, L., P. Sleight, G. Bandinelli, S. Cencetti, L. Fattorini, J. Wdowczyc-Szulc, and A. Lagi. 2001. Effect of rosary prayer and yoga mantras on autonomic cardiovascular rhythms: Comparative study. *British Medical Journal* 323:1446.

Blumenthal, J. A., W. Jang, M. A. Babyak, D. S. Krantz, D. J. Frid, R. E. Coleman, R. Waugh, M. Hanson, M. Applebaum, C. O'Connor, and J. J. Morris. 1997. Stress management and exercise training in cardiac patients with myocardial ischemia. *Archives of Internal Medicine* 157:2213–23.

Brosschot, J. F., and J. F. Thayer. 1998. Anger inhibition, cardiovascular recovery, and vagal function: A model of the link between hostility and cardiovascular disease. *Annals of Behavioral Medicine* 20:326–32.

Brundtland, G. H. 1999. Health for the Twenty-First Century. Speech at the World Economic Forum, January 30, Davos, Switzerland.

Bunker, S. J., D. M. Colquhoun, M. D. Esler, I. B. Hickie, D. Hunt, V. M. Jelinek, B. F. Oldenberg, H. G. Peach, D. Ruth, C. C. Tennat, and A. M. Tonkin. 2003. "Stress" and coronary heart disease: Psychosocial risk factors. National Heart Foundation of Australia Position Statement Update. *Medical Journal of Australia* 178:272–76.

Burell, G. 1996. Behavior medicine interventions in secondary prevention of coronary heart disease. In *Behavioral Medicine Approaches to Cardiovascular Disease Prevention*, edited by K. Orth-Gomer and N. Schneiderman. Mahwah, N.J.: Lawrence Erlbaum.

Burell, G., A. Öhman, Ö. Sundin, G. Ström, B. Ramund, I. Culled, and C. E. Thoresen. 1994. Modification of the type A behavior pattern in post–myocardial infarction patients: A route to cardiac rehabilitation. *International Journal of Behavioral Medicine* 1:32–54.

Carels, R. A., D. Musher-Eizenman, H. Cacciapaglia, C. I. Pérez-Benítez, S. Cristie, and W. O'Brien. 2004. Psychosocial functioning and physical symptoms in heart failure patients: A within-individual approach. *Journal of Psychosomatic Research* 56:95–101.

Carney, R. M., K. E. Freedland, S. Eisen, M. W. Rich, and A. S. Jaffe. 1995. Major depression and medication adherence in elderly patients with coronary artery disease. *Health Psychology* 14:88–90.

Carney, R. M., K. E. Freedland, G. E. Miller, and A. S. Jaffe. 2002. Depression as a risk factor for cardiac mortality and morbidity: A review of potential mechanisms. *Journal of Psychosomatic Research* 53:897–902.

Carney, R. M., K. E. Freedland, P. K. Stein, J. A. Skala, P. Hoffman, and A. S. Jaffe. 2000. Change in heart rate and heart rate variability during treatment for depression in patients with coronary heart disease. *Psychosomatic Medicine* 62:639–47.

Chang, P. P., D. E. Ford, L. A. Meoni, N. Wang, and M. J. Klag. 2002. Anger in young men and subsequent premature cardiovascular disease. *Archives of Internal Medicine* 162:901–6.

Cole, P. A., C. S. Pomerleau, and J. K. Harris. 1993. The effects of noncurrent and concurrent relaxation training on cardiovascular reactivity to a psychological stressor. *Journal of Behavioral Medicine* 15:407–14.

Crowne, J. M., J. Runions, L. S. Ebbesen, N. B. Oldridge, and D. L. Steiner. 1996. Anxiety and depression after acute myocardial infarction. *Heart and Lung* 25:98–107.

Davison, G. C., M. E. Williams, E. Nezami, and T. Bice. 1992. Relaxation, reduction in angry articulated thoughts, and improvements in borderline hypertension and heart rate. *Journal of Behavioral Medicine* 14:453–68.

Del Vecchio, T., and K. D. O'Leary. 2004. Effectiveness of anger treatments for specific anger problems: A meta-analytic review. *Clinical Psychology Review* 24:15–34.

Denollet, J., and D. L. Brutsaert. 2001. Reducing emotional distress improves prognosis in coronary heart disease. *Circulation* 104:2018–23.

Dimidjian, S., and M. M. Linehan. 2003. Mindfulness practice. In *Cognitive Behavior Therapy: Applying Empirically Supported Techniques in Your Practice*, edited by W. O'Donohue, J. E. Fisher, and S. C. Hayes. New York: Wiley.

Dunbar, S. B., L. S. Jenkins, M. Hawthorne, L. P. Kimble, W. N. Dudley, M. Slemmons, and J. A. Purcell. 1999. Factors associated with outcomes 3 months after implantable cardioverter defibrillator insertion. *Heart and Lung* 28:303–15.

D'Zurilla, T. J., and A. M. Nezu. 1999. *Problem-Solving Therapy: A Social Competence Approach to Clinical Intervention.* 2nd ed. New York: Springer.

D'Zurilla, T. J., A. M. Nezu, and A. Maydeu-Olivares. 2004. Social problem solving: Theory and assessment. In *Social Problem Solving: Theory, Research, and Training*, edited by E. C. Chang, T. J. D'Zurilla, and L. J. Sanna. Washington, D.C.: American Psychological Association.

Eaker, E. D., J. Pinsky, and W. P. Castelli. 1992. Myocardial infarction and coronary death among women: Psychosocial predictors from a 20-year follow-up of women in the Framingham Study. *American Journal of Epidemiology* 135:854–64.

Eaker, E. D., L. M. Sullivan, M. Kelly-Hayes, R. B. D'Agostino, and E. J. Benjamin. 2004. Anger and hostility predict the development of atrial fibrillation in men in the Framingham Offspring Study. *Circulation* 109:1267–71.

Edelman, S., J. Lemon, and A. Kidman. 2003. The perceived benefits of a group CBT intervention for patients with coronary heart disease. *Journal of Cognitive Psychotherapy* 17:59–65.

Eller, L. 1999. Guided imagery interventions for symptom management. *Annual Review of Nursing Research* 17:57–84.

Emmons, R. A., and M. E. McCullough. 2003. Counting blessings versus burdens: An experimental investigation of gratitude and subjective well-being in daily life. *Journal of Personality and Social Psychology* 84:377–89.

Enright, R. D. 2001. *Forgiveness Is a Choice: A Step-by-Step Process for Resolving Anger and Restoring Hope.* Washington, D.C.: American Psychological Association.

Enright, R. D., and R. P. Fitzgibbons. 2000. *Helping Clients Forgive: An Empirical Guide for Resolving Anger and Restoring Hope.* Washington, D.C.: American Psychological Association.

Everson, S. A., J. Kauhanen, G. A. Kaplan, D. E. Goldberg, J. Julkunen, J. Tuomilehto, and J. T. Salonen. 1997. Hostility and increased risk of mortality and acute myocardial infarction: The mediating role of behavioral risk factors. *American Journal of Epidemiology* 146:142–52.

Ewart, C. K. 1990. A social problem-solving approach to behavior change in coronary heart disease. In *The Handbook of Health Behavior Change*, edited by S. A. Shumaker. New York: Springer.

Ferguson, K. E. 2003. Relaxation. In *Cognitive Behavior Therapy: Applying Empirically Supported Techniques in Your Practice*, edited by W. O'Donohue, J. E. Fisher, and S. C. Hayes. New York: Wiley.

Fleet, R., K. Lavoie, and B. D. Beitman. 2000. Is panic disorder associated with coronary artery disease? *Journal of Psychosomatic Research* 48:347–56.

Ford, D. E., L. A. Mead, P. P. Chang, L. Cooper-Patrick, N. Wang, and M. J. Klag. 1998. Depression is a risk factor for coronary artery disease in men. *Archives of Internal Medicine* 158:1422–26.

Fors, E. A., H. Sexton, and K. G. Götestam. 2002. The effect of guided imagery and amitriptyline on daily fibromyalgia pain: A prospective, randomized, controlled trial. *Journal of Psychiatric Research* 36:179–87.

Frasure-Smith, N., and F. Lespérance. 2003. Depression and other psychological risks following myocardial infarction. *Archives of General Psychiatry* 60:627–36.

Frasure-Smith, N., F. Lespérance, G. Gravel, A. Masson, M. Juneau, M. Talajic, and M. G. Bourassa. 2000. Depression and health-care costs during the first year following myocardial infarction. *Journal of Psychosomatic Research* 48:471–78.

Frasure-Smith, N., F. Lespérance, and M. Talajic. 1993. Depression following myocardial infarction: Impact on 6-month survival. *Journal of the American Medical Association* 270:1819–25.

Frasure-Smith, N., F. Lespérance, and M. Talajic. 1995. The impact of negative emotions on prognosis following myocardial infarction: Is it more than depression? *Health Psychology* 14:388–98.

Frasure-Smith, N., and R. Prince. 1985. The ischemic heart disease life stress monitoring program: Impact on mortality. *Psychosomatic Medicine* 47:431–45.

Fredrickson, B. L., K. E. Maynard, M. J. Helms, T. L. Haney, I. C. Siegler, and J. C. Barefoot. 2000. Hostility predicts magnitude and duration of blood pressure response to anger. *Journal of Behavioral Medicine* 23:229–43.

Gabbay, F. H., D. S. Krantz, W. J. Kop, S. M. Hedges, J. Klein, J. S. Gottdiener, and A. Rozanski. 1996. Triggers of myocardial ischemia during daily life in patients with coronary artery disease: Physical and mental activities, anger and smoking. *Journal of the American College of Cardiology* 27:585–92.

Gallacher, J. E. J., J. W. G. Yarnell, P. M. Sweetham, P. C. Elwood, and S. A. Stansfeld. 1999. Anger and incident heart disease in the Caerphilly Study. *Psychosomatic Medicine* 61:446–53.

Garcia, L., M. Valdes, I. Inmaculada, and N. Riesco. 1994. Psychological factors and vulnerability to psychiatric morbidity after myocardial infarction. *Psychotherapy and Psychosomatics* 61:187–94.

Gentry, W. D. 2000. *Anger-Free: Ten Basic Steps to Managing Your Anger.* New York: HarperCollins.

Gidron, Y., K. Davidson, and I. Bata. 1999. The short-term effects of a hostility-reduction intervention on male coronary heart disease patients. *Health Psychology* 18:416–20.

Gilbert, C. 2003. Clinical applications of breathing regulation: Beyond anxiety management. *Behavior Modification* 27:692–709.

Goleman, D. 2003. Finding happiness: Cajole your brain to lean to the left. *New York Times,* February 4, F5.

Goodman, M., J. Quigley, G. Moran, H. Meilman, and M. Sherman. 1996. Hostility predicts restenosis after percutaneous transluminal coronary angioplasty. *Mayo Clinic Proceedings* 71:729–34.

Gorman, J. M., and R. P. Sloan. 2000. Depression as a risk factor for cardiovascular and cerebrovascular disease: Emerging data and clinical perspectives. *American Heart Journal* 140:S77–83.

Greenberger, D., and C. Padesky. 1995. *Mind Over Mood: Change How You Feel by Changing the Way You Think.* New York: Guilford Press.

Gross, J. J., and R. W. Levenson. 1997. Hiding feelings: The acute effects of inhibiting negative and positive emotions. *Journal of Abnormal Psychology* 106:95–103.

Haaga, D. A. F., G. C. Davison, M. E. Williams, S. L. Dolezal, J. Haleblian, J. Rosenbaum, J. H. Dwyer, S. Baker, and V. DeQuattro. 1994. Mode-specific impact of relaxation training for hypertensive men with Type A behavior pattern. *Behavior Therapy* 25:209–23.

Hahn, Y. B., Y. J. Ro, H. H. Song, N. C. Kim, H. S. Kim, and Y. S. Yoo. 1994. The effect of thermal biofeedback and progressive muscle relaxation training in reducing blood pressure of patients with essential hypertension. *Image—The Journal of Nursing Scholarship* 25:204–7.

Haines, A. P., J. D. Imeson, and T. W. Meade. 1987. Phobic anxiety and ischemic heart disease. *British Medical Journal* 295:297–99.

Hanh, T. N. 1999. *The Heart of the Buddha's Teaching*. New York: Broadway Books.

Harris, C. R. 2001. Cardiovascular responses of embarrassment and effects of emotional suppression in a social setting. *Journal of Personality and Social Psychology* 81:886–97.

Haugen, N. S. 2000. The effect of autogenic relaxation on hostility and cardiovascular reactivity in African-American women. *Dissertation Abstracts International: Section B: The Sciences and Engineering* 61(6-B):2988.

Hayes, S., K. Strosahl, and K. Wilson. 1999. *Acceptance and Commitment Therapy: An Experiential Approach to Behavior Change*. New York: Guilford Press.

Hayward, C. 1995. Psychiatric illness and cardiovascular disease risk. *Epidemiologic Reviews* 17:129–38.

Hecker, H. M., M. A. Chesney, G. W. Black, and N. Frautschi. 1988. Coronary-prone behavior in the Western Collaborative Group Study. *Psychosomatic Medicine* 50:153–64.

Heller, S., M. Ormont, L. Lidagoster, R. Sciacca, and J. Steinberg. 1998. Psychosocial outcome after ICD implantation: A current perspective. *Pacing and Clinical Electrophysiology* 12:1207–15.

Helmers, K., D. Krantz, R. Howell, J. Klein, N. Bairey, and A. Rozanski. 1993. Hostility and myocardial ischemia in coronary artery disease patients: Evaluation by gender and ischemic index. *Psychosomatic Medicine* 50:29–36.

Hollon, S. D., R. J. DeRubeis, and M. E. P. Seligman. 1992. Cognitive therapy and the prevention of depression. *Applied and Preventative Psychiatry* 95:52–59.

Jacobson, N. S., C. R. Martell, and S. Dimidjian. 2001. Behavioral activation for the treatment of depression: Returning to contextual roots. *Clinical Psychology: Science and Practice* 8:255–70.

Jain, D., T. Joska, F. A. Lee, M. Burg, R. Lampert, and B. L. Zaret. 2001. Day-to-day reproducibility of mental stress–induced abnormal left ventricular function response in patients with coronary artery disease and its relationship to autonomic activation. *Journal of Nuclear Cardiology* 8:347–55.

Jiang, W., M. A. Babyak, A. Rozanski, A. Sherwood, C. M. O'Connor, R. A. Waugh, R. E. Coleman, M. W. Hanson, J. J. Morris, and J. A. Blumenthal. 2002. Depression and increased myocardial ischemic activity in patients with ischemic heart disease. *American Heart Journal* 146:55–61.

Julkumen, J., R. Salomen, G. A. Caplan, M. A. Chesney, and J. T. Salomen. 1994. Hostility and the progression of carotid atherosclerosis. *Psychosomatic Medicine* 56:519–25.

Kabat-Zinn, J. 1995. *Wherever You Go, There You Are: Mindfulness Meditation in Everyday Life.* New York: Hyperion.

Kabat-Zinn, J., L. Lipworth, and R. Burney. 1985. The clinical use of mindfulness meditation for the self-regulation of chronic pain. *Journal of Behavioral Medicine* 8:163–90.

Kawachi, I., G. A. Colditz, A. Ascherio, E. B. Rimm, E. Giovanncucci, M. J. Stampfer, and W. C. Willet. 1994. Prospective study of phobic anxiety and risk of coronary heart disease in men. *Circulation* 89:1992–97.

Kawachi, I., D. Sparrow, A. Spiro, P. Vokonas, and T. Weiss. 1996. A prospective study of anger and coronary heart disease. The Normative Aging Study. *Circulation* 94:2090–95.

Kawachi, I., D. Sparrow, P. S. Vokonas, and S. T. Weiss. 1994. Symptoms of anxiety and risk of coronary heart disease: The Normative Aging Study. *Circulation* 90:2225-29.

Kawachi, I., D. Sparrow, P. S. Vokonas, and S. T. Weiss. 1995. Decreased heart rate variability in men with phobic anxiety. *American Journal of Cardiology* 75:882–85.

Keefe, F. J., P. J. Castell, and J. A. Blumenthal. 1986. Angina pectoris in Type A and type B cardiac patients. *Pain* 27:211-18.

King, M., A. G. Mainous, T. E. Steyer, and W. Pearson. 2001. The relationship between attendance at religious services and cardiovascular inflammatory markers. *International Journal of Psychiatry in Medicine* 31:415–25.

Kivimäki, M., P. Leino-Arjas, R. Luukkonen, H. Riihimäki, J. Vahtera, and J. Kirjonen. 2002. Work stress and risk of cardiovascular mortality: Prospective cohort study of industrial employees. *British Journal of Medicine* 325:325–29.

Koenig, H. G. 1997. *Is Religion Good for Your Health? The Effects of Religion on Physical and Mental Health.* Binghamton, N.Y.: Haworth Pastoral Press.

Koenig, H. G., L. K. George, J. C. Hays, D. B. Larson, H. J. Cohen, and D. G. Blazer. 1998. The relationship between religious activities and blood pressure in older adults. *International Journal of Psychiatry in Medicine* 28:189–213.

Koskenvuo, M., J. Kaprio, R. J. Rose, A. Kesaniemi, S. Sama, K. Heikkila, and H. Langinvaninio. 1988. Hostility as a risk factor for mortality and ischemic heart disease in men. *Psychosomatic Medicine* 50:330–40.

Kubzansky, L. D., I. Kawachi, S. T. Weiss, and D. Sparrow. 1998. Anxiety and coronary heart disease: A synthesis of epidemiological, psychological, and experimental evidence. *Annals of Behavioral Medicine* 20:47–58.

Kubzansky, L. D., D. Sparrow, P. Vokonas, and I. Kawachi. 2001. Is the glass half empty or half full? A prospective study of optimism and coronary heart disease in the Normative Aging Study. *Psychosomatic Medicine* 63:910–16.

Lampert, R., T. Joska, M. M. Burg, W. P. Batsford, C. A. McPherson, and D. Jain. 2002. Emotional and physical precipitants of ventricular arrhythmia. *Circulation* 106:1800–1805.

Lane, D., D. Carroll, C. Ring, D. G. Beevers, and Y. H. Gregory. 2002. The prevalence and persistence of depression and anxiety following myocardial infarction. *British Journal of Health Psychology* 7:11–21.

Larkin, K. T., and C. Zayfert. 1996. Anger management training with essential hypertensive patients. *Journal of Behavioral Medicine* 19:415–33.

Lawler, K. A., J. W. Younger, R. L. Piferi, E. Billington, R. Jobe, K. Edmondson, and W. H. Jones. 2003. A change of heart: Cardiovascular correlates of forgiveness in response to interpersonal conflict. *Journal of Behavioral Medicine* 26:373–93.

Lewinsohn, P. M., R. Munoz, M. A. Youngsen, and A. M. Zeiss. 1978. *Control Your Depression.* New York: Simon and Schuster.

Loewe, B., K. Breining, S. Wilke, R. Wellman, S. Zipfel, and W. Eich. 2002. Quantitative and qualitative effects of Feldenkrais, progressive muscle relaxation, and standard medical treatment in patients after acute myocardial infarction. *Psychotherapy Research* 12:179–91.

Lown, B. 1987. Sudden cardiac death: Biobehavioral perspective. *Circulation* 76:1186–96.

Lown, B., R. L. Verrier, and S. H. Rabinowitz. 1977. Neural and psychological mechanisms and the problem of sudden cardiac death. *American Journal of Cardiology* 39:890–902.

Manne, S. 2003. Coping and social support. In *Health Psychology,* edited by A. M. Nezu, C. M. Nezu, and P. A. Geller. New York: Wiley.

Markovitz, J. H., K. A. Matthews, W. B. Kannel, J. L. Cobb, and R. B. D'Agostino. 1993. Psychological predictors of hypertension in the Framingham Study. Is there tension in hypertension? *Journal of the American Medical Association* 270:2439–43.

Markovitz, J. H., K. A. Matthews, R. R. Wing, L. H. Kuller, and E. N. Meilahn. 1991. Psychological, biological and health behavior predictors of blood pressure changes in middle-aged women. *Journal of Hypertension* 9:399–406.

Marlatt, G. A., and J. L. Kristeller. 1999. Mindfulness and meditation. In *Integrating Spirituality into Treatment: Resources for Practitioners*, edited by W. R. Miller. Washington, D.C.: American Psychological Association.

Matthews, K. A., B. B. Gump, K. F. Harris, T. L. Haney, and J. C. Barefoot. 2004. Hostile behaviors predict cardiovascular mortality among men enrolled in the Multiple Risk Factor Intervention Trial. *Circulation* 109:66–70.

McCraty, R., M. Atkinson, W. A. Tiller, G. Rein, and A. Watkins. 1995. The effects of emotions on short term heart rate variability using power spectrum analysis. *American Journal of Cardiology* 76:1089–93.

McCraty, R., M. Atkinson, and D. Tomasino. 2003. Impact of a workplace stress reduction program on blood pressure and emotional health in hypertensive employees. *Journal of Alternative and Complementary Medicine* 9:355–69.

Mendes de Leon, C. F., W. J. Kop, H. B. de Swart, F. W. Bar, and A. P. Appels. 1996. Psychosocial characteristics and recurrent events after percutaneous transluminal coronary angioplasty. *American Journal of Cardiology* 77:252–55.

Miller, T. Q., T. W. Smith, C. W. Turner, M. L. Guijarro, and A. J. Hallet. 1996. A meta-analytic review of research on hostility and physical health. *Psychological Bulletin* 119:322–48.

Mittleman, M. A., M. Maclure, J. B. Sherwood, R. P. Mulry, G. H. Tofler, S. C. Jacobs, R. Friedman, H. Benson, and J. E. Muller. 1995. Triggering of acute myocardial infarction onset by episodes of anger. *Circulation* 92:1720–25.

Möller, J., J. Hallqvist, F. Diderichsen, T. Theorell, C. Reuterwall, and A. Ahlbom. 1999. Do episodes of anger trigger myocardial infarction? A case-crossover analysis in the Stockholm Heart Epidemiology Program (SHEEP). *Psychosomatic Medicine* 61:842–49.

Morris, E. L. 2001. The relationship of spirituality to coronary heart disease. *Alternative Therapies in Health and Medicine* 7:96–98.

Moser, D. K., and K. Dracup. 1996. Is anxiety early after myocardial infarction associated with subsequent ischemic and arrhythmic events? *Psychosomatic Medicine* 58:395–401.

Mueller, P. S., D. J. Plevak, and T. A. Rummans. 2001. Religious involvement, spirituality, and medicine: Implications for clinical practice. *Mayo Clinic Proceedings* 76:1225–35.

Murberg, T. A., G. Furze, and E. Bru. 2004. Avoidance coping styles predict mortality among patients with congestive heart failure: A 6-year follow-up study. *Personality and Individual Differences* 36:757–66.

Musselman, D. L., D. L. Evans, and C. B. Nemeroff. 1998. The relationship of depression to cardiovascular disease. *Archives of General Psychiatry* 55:580–92.

Musselman, D. L., A. Tomer, A. K. Manatunga, B. T. Knight, M. R. Porter, M. de Baets, U. Marzec, L. A. Harker, and C. B. Nemeroff. 1996. Exaggerated platelet reactivity in major depression. *American Journal of Psychiatry* 153:1212–17.

National Institute of Mental Health. 2004. Anxiety disorders. www.nimh.nih.gov.

Newman, C. 2003. Cognitive restructuring: Identifying and modifying maladaptive schemas. In *Cognitive Behavior Therapy: Applying Empirically Supported Techniques in Your Practice,* edited by W. O'Donohue, J. E. Fisher, and S. C. Hayes. New York: Wiley.

Nezu, A. M. 2004. Problem solving and behavior therapy revisited. *Behavior Therapy* 35:1–33.

Nezu, A. M., C. M. Nezu, and S. E. Blissett. 1988. Sense of humor as a moderator of the relation between stressful events and psychological distress: A prospective analysis. *Journal of Personality and Social Psychology* 54:520–25.

Nezu, A. M., C. M. Nezu, S. H. Felgoise, K. S. McClure, and P. S. Houts. 2003. Project Genesis: Assessing the efficacy of problem-solving therapy for distressed adult cancer patients. *Journal of Consulting and Clinical Psychology* 71:1036–48.

Nezu, A. M., C. M. Nezu, S. H. Friedman, S. Faddis, and P. S. Houts. 1998. *Helping Cancer Patients Cope: A Problem-Solving Approach.* Washington, D.C.: American Psychological Association.

Nezu, A. M., C. M. Nezu, and P. A. Geller, eds. 2003. *Health Psychology.* New York: Wiley.

Nezu, A. M., C. M. Nezu, D. Jain, V. M. Wilkins, and M. A. Shepanski. 2004. Depression and Cardiovascular Disease. Paper presented at the annual scientific convention of the Association for Advancement of Behavior Therapy, New Orleans.

Nezu, A. M., C. M. Nezu, and E. R. Lombardo. 2001. Cognitive-behavior therapy for medically unexplained symptoms: A critical review of the treatment literature. *Behavior Therapy* 32:537–83.

Nezu, A. M., C. M. Nezu, and E. R. Lombardo. 2003. Problem-solving therapy. In *Cognitive Behavior Therapy: Applying Empirically Supported Techniques in Your Practice*, edited by W. O'Donohue, J. E. Fisher, and S. C. Hayes. New York: Wiley.

Nezu, A. M., C. M. Nezu, and E. R. Lombardo. 2004. *Cognitive-Behavioral Case Formulation and Treatment Design: A Problem-Solving Approach*. New York: Springer.

Nezu, A. M., V. M. Wilkins, and C. M. Nezu. 2004. Social problem solving, stress, and negative affective conditions. In *Social Problem Solving: Theory, Research, and Training*, edited by E. C. Chang, T. J. D'Zurilla, and L. J. Sanna. Washington, D.C.: American Psychological Association.

Nezu, C. M., and A. M. Nezu. 2003. *Awakening Self-Esteem: Spiritual and Psychological Techniques to Enhance Your Well-Being*. Oakland, Calif.: New Harbinger.

Ornish, D. 1996. *Dr. Dean Ornish's Program for Reversing Heart Disease*. New York: Ivey Books.

Pearsall, P. 1998. *The Heart's Code: Tapping the Wisdom and Power of Our Heart Energy*. New York: Broadway Books.

Pennebaker, J. W. 1995. *Emotion, Disclosure, and Health*. Washington, D.C.: American Psychological Association.

Peters, R. W., S. McQuillan, S. K. Resnick, and M. R. Gold. 1996. Increased Monday incidence of life-threatening ventricular arrhythmias. *Circulation* 94:1346–49.

Polackova, J., E. Bockova, and V. Sedivec. 1982. Autogenic training: Application in secondary prevention of myocardial infarction. *Activitas Nervosa Superior* 24:178–80.

Rehm, L. P., and J. H. Adams. 2003. Self management. In *Cognitive Behavior Therapy: Applying Empirically Supported Techniques in Your Practice*, edited by W. O'Donohue, J. E. Fisher, and S. C. Hayes. New York: Wiley.

Rosenberg, E. L., P. Ekman, W. Jiang, M. Babyak, R. E. Coleman, M. Hanson, C. O'Connor, R. Waugh, and J. A. Blumenthal. 2001. Linkages between facial expressions of anger and transient myocardial ischemia in men with coronary artery disease. *Emotion* 1:107–15.

Rosenman, R. H., R. J. Brand, C. D. Jenkins, M. Friedman, R. Strauss, and M. Wurm 1975. Coronary heart disease in the Western Collaborative Group Study: Final follow-up experience of 8.5 years. *Journal of the American Medical Association* 223:872–77.

Rossi, N., R. Caldari, F. V. Costa, and E. Ambrosioni. 1989. Autogenic training in mild essential hypertension: A placebo-controlled study. *Stress Medicine* 5:63–68.

Rozanski, A., J. A. Blumenthal, and J. Kaplan. 1999. Impact of psychological factors on the pathogenesis of cardiovascular disease and implications for therapy. *Circulation* 99:2192–217.

Scheier, M. F., K. A. Matthews, J. F. Owens, G. J. McGovern, R. C. Lefebvre, R. A. Abbott, and C. S. Carver. 2003. Dispositional optimism and recovery from coronary artery bypass surgery: The beneficial effects on physical and psychological well-being. In *Social Psychology and Health: Key Readings in Social Psychology*, edited by P. Salovey and A. J. Rothman. New York: Psychology Press.

Schneiderman, N. 1987. Psychophysiologic factors in atherogenesis and coronary artery disease. *Circulation* 76:141–47.

Shapiro, P. A., R. P. Sloan, E. Bagiella, J. P. Kuhl, S. Anjilvel, and J. J. Mann. 2000. Cerebral activation, hostility, and cardiovascular control during mental stress. *Journal of Psychosomatic Research* 48:485–91.

Shen, B. J., C. P. McCreary, and H. F. Myers. 2004. Independent and mediated contributions of personality, coping, social support, and depressive symptoms to physical functioning outcome among patients in cardiac rehabilitation. *Journal of Behavioral Medicine* 27:39–62.

Shiotani, I., H. Sato, K. Kinjo, D. Nakatani, H. Mizuno, Y. Ohnishi, E. Hishida, Y. Kijima, M. Hori, and H. Sato. 2002. Depressive symptoms predict 12-month prognosis in elderly patients with acute myocardial infarction. *Journal of Cardiovascular Risk* 9:153–60.

Sirois, B. C., and M. M. Burg. 2003. Negative emotion and coronary heart disease: A review. *Behavior Modification* 27:83–103.

Skeie, T. M., S. Skeie, and T. C. Stiles. 1989. The effectiveness of pleasant imagery and a distraction task as coping strategies in alleviating experimentally induced dysphoric mood. *Scandinavian Journal of Behavioural Therapy* 18:31–42.

Sloan, R. P., P. A. Shapiro, J. Thomas Bigger, E. Bagiella, R. C. Steinman, and J. M. Gorman. 1994. Cardiac autonomic control and hostility in healthy subjects. *American Journal of Cardiology* 74:298–300.

Smith, T. W., and L. C. Gallo. 1999. Hostility and cardiovascular reactivity during marital interaction. *Psychosomatic Medicine* 61:436–45.

Spiegel, D., and R. Moore. 1997. Imagery and hypnosis in the treatment of cancer patients. *Oncology* 11:1179–89.

Stetter, F., and S. Kupper. 2002. Autogenic training: A meta-analysis of clinical outcome studies. *Applied Psychophysiology and Biofeedback* 27:45–98.

Stoney, C. M. 1998. Coronary heart disease. In *Behavioral Medicine and Women: A Comprehensive Handbook*, edited by E. A. Blechman and K. D. Brownell. New York: Guilford.

Stowell, J. R., L. McGuire, T. Robles, R. Glaser, and J. K. Kiecolt-Glaser. 2003. Psychoneuroimmunology. In *Health Psychology*, edited by A. M. Nezu, C. M. Nezu, and P. A. Geller. New York: Wiley.

Suarez, E. C., and J. A. Blumenthal. 1991. Ambulatory blood pressure responses during daily life in high and low hostile patients with a recent myocardial infarction. *Journal of Cardiopulmonary Rehabilitation* 11:169–75.

Sudsuang, R., V. Chentanez, and K. Veluvan. 1991. Effect of Buddhist meditation on serum cortisol and total protein levels, blood pressure, pulse rate, lung volume and reaction time. *Physiology and Behavior* 50:543–48.

Sul, J., and C. K. Wan. 1993. The relationship between trait hostility and cardiovascular reactivity: A quantitative analysis. *Psychophysiology* 30:615–26.

Teasdale, J. D., Z. V. Segal, J. M. Williams, V. A. Ridgeway, J. M. Saulsy, and M. A. Lace. 2000. Prevention of relapse/recurrence in major depression by mindfulness-based cognitive therapy. *Journal of Consulting and Clinical Psychology* 68:615–23.

Thomas, S. A., E. Friedman, M. Khatta, L. C. Cook, and A. L. Lann. 2003. Depression in patients with heart failure: Physiologic effects, incidence, and relation to mortality. *AACN Clinical Issues* 14:3–12.

Thoreson, C. E., and P. Bracke. 1997. Reducing coronary recurrences and coronary-prone behavior: A structured group treatment approach. In *Group Therapy for Medically Ill Patients*, edited by J. L. Spira. New York: Guilford.

Vaccarino, V., S. V. Kasal, J. Abramson, and H. M. Krumholz. 2001. Depressive symptoms and risk of functional decline and death in patients with heart failure. *Journal of the American College of Cardiology* 38:199–205.

Vogt, T. M., J. P. Mullooly, D. Ernst, C. R. Pope, and J. F. Hollis. 1992. Social networks as predictors of ischemic heart disease, cancer, stroke, and hypertension: Incidence, survival, and mortality. *Journal of Clinical Epidemiology* 45:659–66.

Walton, K. G., R. H. Schneider, S. I. Nidich, J. W. Salerno, C. K. Nordstrom, and C. N. B. Merz. 2002. Psychosocial stress and cardiovascular disease. Part 2: Effectiveness of the Transcendental Meditation program in treatment and prevention. *Behavioral Medicine* 28:106–23.

Watkins, L. L., P. Grossman, R. Krishnan, and A. Sherwood. 1998. Anxiety and vagal control of heart rate. *Psychosomatic Medicine* 60:498–502.

Weil, A. 1996. *Spontaneous Healing: How to Discover and Embrace Your Body's Natural Ability to Maintain and Heal Itself*. New York: Ballantine Books.

Wenzlaff, R. M., and D. M. Wegner. 2002. Thought suppression. *Annual Review of Psychology* 51:59–91.

Williams, R. B., J. C. Barefoot, and R. M. Califf. 1992. Prognostic importance of social and economic resources among medically treated patients with angiographically demonstrated coronary artery disease. *Journal of the American Medical Association* 267:520–24.

Wills, T. A. 1998. Social support. In *Behavioral Medicine and Women: A Comprehensive Handbook,* edited by E. A. Blechman and K. D. Brownell. New York: Guilford.

Witvliet, C., T. E. Ludwig, and K. L. Vander Laan. 2001. Granting forgiveness and harboring grudges: Implications for emotion, physiology, and health. *Psychological Science* 121:117–23.

Wulsin, L. R., and B. M. Singal. 2003. Do depressive symptoms increase the risk for the onset of coronary disease? A systematic quantitative review. *Psychosomatic Medicine* 65:201–10.

Zamarra, J. W., R. H. Schneider, I. Besseghini, D. K. Robinson, and J. W. Salerno. 1996. Usefulness of the Transcendental Meditation program in the treatment of patients with coronary artery disease. *American Journal of Cardiology* 77:867–70.

About the Authors

Arthur M. Nezu, Ph.D., ABPP, professor of psychology, medicine, and public health, is codirector of the Center for Behavioral Medicine and Mind/Body Studies at Drexel University. He is past president of the Association for Advancement of Behavior Therapy, the World Congress of Behavioural and Cognitive Therapies, the Behavioral Psychology Specialty Council, and currently president of the American Board of Behavioral and Cognitive Psychology. Dr. Nezu is a fellow of the American Psychological Association, the American Psychological Society, the Society of Behavioral Medicine, the American Academy of Behavioral and Cognitive Psychology, and the Academy of Cognitive Therapy.

Christine Maguth Nezu, Ph.D., ABPP, professor of psychology and associate professor of medicine, is codirector of the Center for Behavioral Medicine and Mind/Body Studies at Drexel University. She is currently on the board of trustees of the American Board of Professional Psychology as well as on the board of directors of the American Board of Behavioral and Cognitive Psychology. Dr. Maguth Nezu is a fellow of the American Academy of Behavioral and Cognitive Psychology and the Academy of Cognitive Therapy.

Diwakar Jain, MD, FACC, FRCP, is professor of cardiovascular medicine and director of nuclear cardiology at Drexel University College of Medicine. He is currently on the board of directors of the American Society of Nuclear Cardiology. Dr. Jain is a fellow of the American College of Cardiology and the Royal College of Physicians.